# ETHNICITY, CLASS AND HEALTH

---

## JAMES Y NAZROO

is Reader in Sociology and head of the Health and Social Surveys Research Group in the Department of Epidemiology, UCL. He was previously a Research Fellow in the Department of Social Policy and Social Sciences at Royal Holloway, and a Senior Research Fellow in PSI's Ethnic Equality and Diversity Group. His other publications include *Ethnic Minorities in Britain* (*et al*, PSI, 1997), *The Health of Britain's Ethnic Minorities* (PSI, 1997) and *Ethnicity and Mental Health* (PSI, 1997).

# Ethnicity, Class and Health

JAMES Y NAZROO

Policy Studies Institute

UNIVERSITY OF WESTMINSTER

*PSI is a wholly owned subsidiary of the University of Westminster*

ISBN 0 85374 792  X
PSI Report No. 880

Cover design by Andrew Corbett
Typeset by PCS Mapping & DTP, Newcastle upon Tyne
Printed by Athenaeum Press Ltd

Policy Studies Institute
For further information contact
Publications Dept, PSI, 100 Park Village East, London NW1 3SR
Tel (020) 7468 0468   Fax (020) 7468 2211   Email pubs@psi.org.uk

# Contents

# Tables and Figures

# Acronyms and Abbreviations

| | |
|---|---|
| CHD | coronary heart disease |
| CIS-R | Clinical Interview Schedule |
| d.f. | degrees of freedom |
| ECG | electrocardiogram |
| GP | general practitioner |
| ICD | International Classification of Disease |
| MRC | Medical Research Council |
| NHS | National Health Service |
| OPCS | Office for Population Censuses and Surveys |
| PSE | Present State Examination |
| PSQ | Psychosis Screening Questionnaire |
| SCAN | Schedules for Clinical Assessment in Neuropsychiatry |
| UK | United Kingdom |
| US | United States of America |
| WHO | World Health Organisation |

# Preface

The initial analyses of the Fourth National Survey of Ethnic Minorities were presented in three volumes published in 1997 by the Policy Studies Institute: *Ethnic Minorities in Britain: Diversity and Disadvantage*, *The Health of Britain's Ethnic Minorities*, and *Ethnicity and Mental Health*. This volume brings together the two publications on health, integrating, revising and updating them, and using insights and findings from secondary analyses of the Fourth National Survey. In this revised volume, the focus is on explanation rather than description. So, the emphasis here is to examine critically and test the utility of various approaches to understanding ethnic differences in health, using both the mental and physical health data from the Fourth National Survey. It is argued that we cannot fully understand the relationship between ethnicity and health without adequately and explicitly theorising ethnicity, and that conceptualising ethnic differences in health as *inequalities* in health requires careful consideration of the relationship between 'race', ethnicity and class. It is this task that this volume sets out to begin to address.

Chapter 1 sets the context for this volume. It describes the make-up and situation of the ethnic minority population in England and Wales. It then goes on to examine critically existing evidence on ethnic differences in health and explanations for them, with a particularly close examination of the contested evidence on ethnic differences in mental health. Chapter 2 describes the methods used in the conduct of the Fourth National Survey, in particular sampling strategies and approaches to the measurement of both ethnicity and health. Particular attention is given to the difficulties inherent in a cross-cultural exploration of differences in mental health, with some detail provided on the innovative approaches to the assessment of mental health used here. Chapter 3 provides basic data on differences in health across the ethnic groups included in the Fourth National Survey. It covers a number of key health outcomes: general health; long-standing illness; cardiovascular disease (coronary heart disease and hypertension); diabetes; respiratory disease; smoking; neurotic depression; and non-affective psychosis, and provides both absolute rates of illness within ethnic groups, by gender, and the relative risk of illness for ethnic minority groups compared with the white group. Chapters

4 and 5 extend the critical examination of the concept of ethnicity by examining how far the emergent ethnic differences in health described in Chapter 3 might be consistent across ethnic sub-groups (Chapter 4 examines this in terms of religious sub-groups for the Indian or African Asian ethnic grouping) and across generations (Chapter 5 examines this in terms of age on migration to the UK). Chapter 5 also uses the findings on the relationship between ethnic differences in mental health, age on migration and fluency in English to examine the possibility that the western conceptualisation of mental health does not adequately cover the experiences of other cultural groups.

Chapter 6 provides the examination of socio-economic effects that is central to this volume. It begins by using traditional indicators of socio-economic position to illustrate the presence of class gradients in health within ethnic groups. It then discusses conceptual and methodological problems with attempts to assess the contribution of socio-economic effects to inequalities in health across ethnic groups. It moves on to develop an index of socio-economic position, derived from the depth of contextual information uniquely available in the Fourth National Survey, and to use this index to explore the contribution of socio-economic effects to ethnic inequalities in health. Chapter 7 provides a summary of the findings presented in earlier chapters. It then goes on to examine critically the implications of these findings to an understanding of ethnic inequalities in health, focusing on the need to theorise ethnicity adequately and to tackle the central debate around structure (class and racism) and agency (ethnicity as identity).

# Acknowledgements

This volume is one of a series based on the Fourth National Survey of Ethnic Minorities. The Fourth National Survey was supported and undertaken by several people and organisations. Data collection was jointly sponsored by the Economic and Social Research Council; the Department of Health; the Department of the Environment; the Department for Education and Employment, with the Employment Service; and the Joseph Rowntree Charitable Trust.

The research itself was undertaken in partnership by the Policy Studies Institute and Social and Community Planning Research, who were responsible for survey design, data collection and preparation of the data. At PSI a number of colleagues contributed to the work. David Smith was originally responsible for getting the Fourth National Survey off the ground, and led the team through the design phase, with David Halpern leading the development and design of the health element of the questionnaire. Richard Berthoud then took on overall responsibility for the study, with Sharon Beishon, Tariq Modood and Satnam Virdee all making major contributions to the ideas that informed the analyses presented here.

This work also benefited from advice and comments from a large number of friends and colleagues in universities and research institutes, in government and elsewhere, and this volume owes a great debt to their contributions. I would particularly like to thank my PhD supervisor, Graham Scambler, for his support and invaluable advice during the conduct of this research.

All of these people and organisations contributed to the research. Above all, though, I am grateful to the 8000 people who took part in the survey and provided information about their experiences and opinions.

# CHAPTER ONE

# Introduction

Over the last three decades there has been considerable interest in both class inequalities in health and the health of ethnic minority populations. A relatively early, but key, publication in both of these fields has influenced the direction they took – the Black Report (Townsend and Davidson, 1982) on class inequalities in health and Marmot et al.'s (1984) study of immigrant mortality. Importantly, these two pieces of work came to quite different conclusions. The Black Report placed emphasis on material explanations for the higher risk of morbidity and mortality among poorer class groups, which, given the class locations of ethnic minority people at that time (Brown 1984), would suggest that such issues might also be relevant to ethnic inequalities in health. However, the data published on immigrant mortality rates, a few years after the Black Report, indicated that class and, consequently, material explanations were unrelated to mortality rates for most migrant groups, and made no contribution to the higher mortality rates found among those who had migrated to Britain (Marmot et al., 1984). Indeed, for one group, those born in the 'Caribbean Commonwealth', the relationship between class and overall mortality rates was the opposite of that for the general population, with those in better off class groups having higher rates of mortality. Marmot et al. concluded:

> (a) that differences in social class distribution are not the explanation of the overall different mortality of migrants; and (b) the relation of social class (as usually defined) to mortality is different among immigrant groups from the England and Wales pattern (Marmot et al., 1984: 21).

The two fields have subsequently taken quite different directions. Those interested in class inequalities have, on the whole, concentrated on providing additional evidence for a material explanation and unpacking the mechanisms that might link material disadvantage with a greater risk of poor health (e.g. Lundeberg, 1991; Davey Smith et al., 1994; Vågerö and Illsley, 1995;

Macintyre, 1997). While, with a few notable exceptions (Ahmad et al., 1989; Fenton et al., 1995; Smaje, 1995a; Harding and Maxwell, 1997), class has until recently disappeared from investigations into the relationship between ethnicity and health, particularly in Britain, and the emphasis has been placed on the contribution that cultural or genetic factors might make. For example, in an overview of existing data produced for the NHS Executive and NHS Ethnic Health Unit, there is no mention of class, even though there is some discussion of other demographic features of the ethnic minority population of Britain (Balarajan and Soni Raleigh, 1995).

In contrast to the data published by Marmot et al. (1984), work in the US has suggested both that material factors are relevant to the health of ethnic minority people and that they make the key contribution to differences in health between different ethnic groups (Rogers, 1992; Sterling et al., 1993; Davey Smith et al., 1996 and 1998). But, in some ways findings suggesting a material base for ethnic inequalities in health run counter to the wider sociological literature on ethnicity and 'race'. Although within this work there appears to be complete agreement that 'race' is a concept without scientific validity (see, for example, the collected works in Barot 1996) – an artificial construct, used to justify the hierarchical ordering of groups of people and the exploitation of 'inferior races' – in contrast, most writers give credence to a notion of ethnicity, which reflects self-identification with cultural traditions that both provide strength and meaning, and boundaries (perhaps fluid) between groups. So, although the construction of ethnic or racial categories might have a material base (Miles, 1989) and socio-economic disadvantage might contribute to ethnic inequalities in health, it is suggested that there remains a cultural component to ethnicity that could make a major contribution to differences in health; that when explaining the relationship between ethnicity and health, ethnicity cannot be 'simply emptied into class disadvantage' (Smaje, 1996).

Such discussions do, of course, implicitly raise questions regarding the ontological status of ethnicity (and race), which are rarely addressed in the health literature (see Smaje, 1996, for an exception to this, and Scambler and Higgs, 1999, who develop this point in relation to the operationalisation and discussion of class in the wider literature on inequalities in health), but which are implicit in the types of explanations posited for ethnic differences in health. The analytical framework used within the ethnicity and health literature largely operates from an epidemiological perspective and has been developed from that proposed in the Black Report (Townsend and Davidson, 1982). It typically includes the following range of explanations (derived from Andrews and Jewson, 1993):

• Differences are the result of a statistical artefact resulting from biases in sampling and biases in outcome measurement. Members of ethnic minority groups may be under-counted in the population from which statistics are calculated (under-enumeration in the 1991 Census, for example, is discussed later); and they may be over- or under-counted in the ill group, perhaps as a result of being more or less likely to be treated than equivalent white people, or because members of different ethnic groups may interpret differently and respond differently to the same survey questions about their health (see the discussion in Chapter 2).

- Differences shown in immigrant mortality data could be a consequence of migration effects. Those who were more healthy may have been more likely to migrate, particularly if they had to travel some distance – a 'healthy migrant' effect (Marmot et al., 1984). The process of migration, with associated cultural dislocation and stress, could directly (adversely) affect the health of migrants (Hull, 1979). And the environmental conditions in the country of birth, or the mother's country of birth, may adversely affect the health of an individual.

- Genetic or biological differences in risk might underlie ethnic differences in health.

- Cultural differences, in particular differences in lifestyles, values and beliefs, might contribute to differences in health.

- Experiencing racism might have a direct effect on health, perhaps through psychological mechanisms.

- Poorer access to health care services, or poorer quality of care, might also help explain the poorer health of certain ethnic groups.

- Differences in material circumstances between ethnic groups might contribute, as the Black Report (Townsend and Davidson, 1982) argued they do to class inequalities in health.

Given the existence of such lists, and the favouring of cultural or genetic explanations within them, it is perhaps not surprising that the health literature has been extensively criticised for essentialising both ethnicity and 'race', i.e. treating them as real and explanations in their own right. Within this predominantly epidemiological literature, the crude operationalisation of ethnic/'race' categories (e.g. through assessment of country of birth, or interviewers' observations, or, more recently, the adaption of the 1991 Census question) is assumed to reflect real and homogeneous biological or cultural groupings, with explanations consequently based on unmeasured stereotyped assumptions of cultural or genetic difference (Sheldon and Parker, 1992; Ahmad, 1993b). Of course, from an epidemiological perspective, how a disease is socially patterned provides important clues for an investigation of its aetiology. So, studies exploring variations in disease patterns across ethnic groups can, by focusing on the attributes of those at greater risk of an adverse outcome, be used to provide an understanding of aetiology (the way in which this rationale underlies health research can be clearly seen in the work of Marmot et al., (1984) and McKeigue and colleagues (e.g. McKeigue et al., 1988, 1989 and 1991)). Unfortunately, this is done with crudely conceptualised ethnic groupings and an almost inevitable focus on the unmeasured, or indirectly measured, genetic or cultural characteristics of individuals within ethnic minority groups, who then become pathologised (Ahmad, 1993b; Sashidharan and Francis, 1993). (Krieger, 1994, provides a useful critique of this traditional epidemiological approach; Arber, 1990, discusses this in relation to gender inequalities in health; and Bhopal, 1997, applies the critique of this 'Black Box' approach to epidemiological work on ethnicity.) This can then lead to an extension of the racialisation of the ethnic minority category under investigation.

In contrast, as described above, the sociological literature on ethnicity has, to a large extent, focused on ethnicity as identity and, as such, has mirrored the anti-essentialism found in work on identity more generally (Modood, 1998). So, here ethnicity is conceived of as 'a shifting category which can change over time, whether defined by individuals themselves or others' (Hillier and Kelleher, 1996: 2). While ethnicity is considered to reflect identification with sets of shared values, beliefs, customs and lifestyles, it has to be understood dynamically, as an active social process (Smaje, 1996). In particular, the influence of the culture of individuals and groups on their health has to be properly contextualised. The emphasis is on agency and the construction of identity, but, as the above quote from Hillier and Kelleher (1996) suggests, it acknowledges power relations and social structure as well.

Of course, as with any attempt to provide a sociological understanding, it is important to consider ethnicity as both agency and structure. Miles writes:

> the category of 'ethnic' and its various derivatives ... is not so much a matter of cultural difference *per se* as one of employing a conception of difference (which may or may not have a 'real' object) to negotiate and sustain a boundary within a wider set of social relations. In other words, the 'ethnic moment' occurs when a claim to a distinct origin, history, and 'mode of being' in the social world can distinguish and mobilise (actively or passively) a supra-class and gender divided social collectivity, and always in relation to another or to a multiplicity of others. Ethnic phenomena are therefore relational (including relations of inclusion and exclusion) and political. But they are not autonomous: by occurring always within a wider set of social relations (that is within, for the past five centuries, an evolving world capitalist economy which has been divided politically into discrete fields of political domination), the organisation and effects of ethnic collectivities are mediated through the political economy of this evolution (Miles, 1996: 252–3).

Miles suggests that the construction of ethnic boundaries is economically determined, but, regardless of this, his comments are a reminder both that ethnic identity is assigned as well as adopted (and assigned on the basis of power relations) and that ethnic minority status is closely associated with particular class positions.

Not surprisingly, the necessarily crude operationalisaton of ethnicity in large-scale quantitative surveys, including the one to be reported on here, does not adequately deal with either issues relating to ethnicity as agency (adopted identity) or ethnicity as structure (the relational nature of ethnicity). These issues will be returned to throughout this volume, but here, before going on to discuss the literature on ethnic differences in health in more detail, some recent evidence on the lives of ethnic minority people in Britain will first be summarised.

## ETHNIC MINORITY GROUPS IN BRITAIN

In order to set the context for this volume, this section will provide a brief description of the ethnic minority population of Britain, predominantly covering demographics. Most of what we know about the social and economic circumstances of the ethnic minority population of Britain comes from the 1991 Census (Coleman and Salt, 1996; Peach, 1996; Ratcliffe, 1996; Karn, 1997) and the Fourth National Survey of Ethnic Minorities (Modood et al., 1997), although data from the 2001 Census will be available shortly.

The 1991 Census included questions on country of birth and, for the first time in a British census, ethnic group. Previously the census had only asked about nationality and country of birth. In 1991 respondents were asked to indicate which ethnic group they belonged to from a fixed range of choices that encompassed both skin colour and country of origin. The original fixed-choice categories covered: White; Black – Caribbean; Black – African; Black – Other (please describe); Indian; Pakistani; Bangladeshi; Chinese; Any Other Ethnic Group (please describe). For those with 'mixed descent', respondents were instructed to use the category that was most appropriate or the 'Any Other Ethnic Group' category together with a description. Responses to the ethnic group question, 'recoded' into ten categories, are shown in Table 1.1, along with the percentage in each group who were born in Britain. The table shows that in 1991 5.5 per cent of the population (just over three million people) identified themselves as belonging to one of the listed ethnic minority groups. Almost half of these people were born in Britain.

The table also shows the diversity of the origins of ethnic minority people in Britain, with the largest group, Indians, making up only just over a quarter of ethnic minority people and some of the groups, including Indians, very obviously encompassing quite diverse sub-groups. When reading this table it is important to note that undercounting at the 1991 Census varied by ethnic group in addition to age and gender. The undercount appeared to be greatest for young ethnic minority men; published adjustment tables suggest that for 25 to 29-year-old ethnic minority men the undercount was in the range of 13 to 17 per cent (OPCS, 1994; Peach, 1996).

Analysis of the 1991 Census has also shown that there were important differences in the geographical locations of different ethnic groups. The ethnic

**Table 1.1    Ethnic composition of the UK population at the 1991 Census**

| Ethnic group | Number | Per cent | Per cent born in UK |
|---|---|---|---|
| White | 51,873,794 | 94.5 | 95.8 |
| All ethnic minorities | 3,015,050 | 5.5 | 46.8 |
| All Black | 890,727 | 1.6 | 55.7 |
|   Black–Caribbean | 499,964 | 0.9 | 53.7 |
|   Black–African | 212,362 | 0.4 | 36.4 |
|   Black–Other[1] | 178,401 | 0.3 | 84.4 |
| All South Asian | 1,479,645 | 2.7 | 44.1 |
|   Indian | 840,255 | 1.5 | 43.0 |
|   Pakistani | 476,555 | 0.9 | 50.5 |
|   Bangladeshi | 162,835 | 0.3 | 36.7 |
| Chinese and others | 644,678 | 1.2 | 40.6 |
|   Chinese | 156,938 | 0.3 | 28.4 |
|   Other–Asian | 197,534 | 0.4 | 21.9 |
|   Other–Other[2] | 290,206 | 0.5 | 59.8 |

1 The 'Black–Other' group contains people recorded as 'Black' with no further details, those identifying themselves as 'Black British', and people with ethnic origins classified as mixed black/white and black/other ethnic group. It seems that most of the 'Black–Other' group had Caribbean family origins, but were born in Britain (Peach, 1996).

2 The 'Other–Other' group contains North Africans, Arabs, Iranians, together with people of mixed Asian/white, mixed Black/white and 'other' mixed categories (Peach, 1996).

minority population is largely concentrated in England and mainly in the most populous areas. Owen's (1992, 1994a) analysis of the 1991 Census data showed that:

- More than half (56.2 per cent) of the ethnic minority population lived in South East England, where less than a third (31.3 per cent) of the total population lived.
- Greater London contained 44.8 per cent of the ethnic minority population and only 10.3 per cent of the total population.
- Elsewhere the West Midlands, West Yorkshire and Greater Manchester displayed the highest relative concentrations of people from ethnic minorities.
- Almost 70 per cent of ethnic minority people lived in Greater London, the West Midlands, West Yorkshire and Greater Manchester, compared with just over 25 per cent of all people.
- There are even greater differences when smaller areas are considered; more than half of ethnic minority people lived in enumeration districts where the total ethnic minority population exceeds 44 per cent, compared with the 5.5 per cent national average.

There are also important differences between the geographical locations of different ethnic minority groups. For example, in the South Asian category

**Table 1.2    Types of areas where ethnic minority and white people live**

*Percentages*

| OPCS classification | White | All ethnic minorities | All black groups | South Asian |
|---|---|---|---|---|
| Established high status | 14.0 | 17.1 | 14.1 | 16.6 |
| Higher status growth | 9.4 | 3.1 | 2.8 | 2.3 |
| More rural areas | 13.1 | 1.6 | 1.4 | 0.6 |
| Resort and retirement | 5.4 | 1.1 | 0.8 | 0.6 |
| Mixed town and country, some industry | 23.3 | 8.3 | 5.7 | 9.3 |
| Traditional manufacturing | 8.4 | 27.8 | 20.0 | 39.2 |
| Service centres and cities | 13.7 | 11.3 | 12.1 | 9.5 |
| Areas with much local authority housing | 8.4 | 4.2 | 2.5 | 5.2 |
| Parts of Inner London | 3.2 | 21.8 | 35.8 | 14.9 |
| Central London | 1.0 | 3.8 | 5.2 | 1.8 |

Indian people are more concentrated in London and the West Midlands, Pakistani people are more concentrated in West Yorkshire, Greater Manchester and the West Midlands, and Bangladeshi people are strongly concentrated in London, Birmingham and Greater Manchester.

Table 1.2, drawn from Owen (1992), uses an Office for Population Censuses and Surveys (OPCS) classification to characterise local authorities and shows the percentage of different ethnic groups living in each type. It clearly shows the higher concentration of white people in rural and suburban areas and the higher concentration of ethnic minority people in industrial areas and London.

There are also differences in the age and gender profiles of different ethnic groups. Differences in gender profiles for different ethnic groups probably reflect differences in the recency and patterns of migration, with men typically migrating first and women and children joining them later. So analysis of the 1991 Census showed that among the South Asian and Black–African groups, males outnumbered females. For the other groups, including whites, there were more women than men (Owen, 1993).

The 1991 Census also showed the relative youth of ethnic minority groups (Owen, 1993). Children formed a third of the ethnic minority population, compared with under a fifth of the white population. In contrast, while 16 per cent of the population as a whole were aged over 65, only just over 3 per cent of the ethnic minority population fell within this age group. Differences in age profiles are summarised in Figure 1.1, which also suggests differences in the age structures of particular ethnic minority groups (for example the South Asian group has a high proportion of people in the 5 to 15 age range). In summary, among the ethnic minority groups Black–Caribbeans, Chinese, Indians and Other Asians tended to be older, while Bangladeshis, Pakistanis and, not surprisingly, Black–Others, were younger.

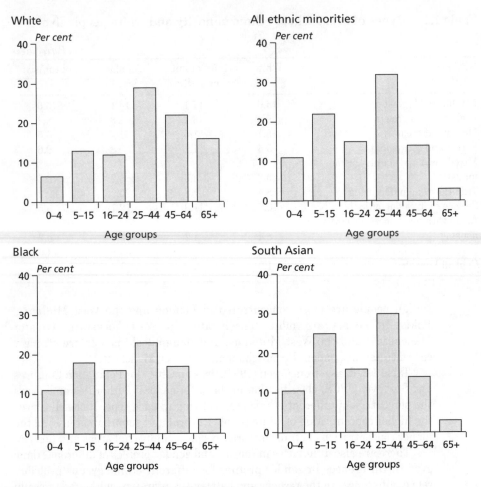

**Figure 1.1   Age profiles for different ethnic groups**

Differences in family formation, household structure and household size across ethnic groups in Britain also exist. Analysis of the 1991 Census (Coleman and Salt, 1996) and the Fourth National Survey (Berthoud and Beishon, 1997) showed that white, Caribbean, Indian and Chinese families had similar numbers of children, while Pakistani and Bangladeshi families had many more children. An analysis of the Fourth National Survey (Berthoud and Beishon, 1997), which took into account life-stage, suggested that most white families would have one or two children and more than 90 per cent of them would have no more than three children. In contrast, most Pakistani and Bangladeshi families would have four or more children and 85 per cent of them would have three or more children. South Asian households were also larger because of the number of adults they contained. Half of Pakistani and Bangladeshi households had three or more adults in them,

**Table 1.3  Household incomes and ethnicity**

*Percentages*

| | White | Caribbean | Indian | Pakistani | Bangladeshi | Chinese |
|---|---|---|---|---|---|---|
| More than $1^{1}/_{2}$ times average | 23 | 12 | 14 | 1 | 2 | 22 |
| $^{1}/_{2}$ to $1^{1}/_{2}$ times average | 49 | 47 | 45 | 17 | 14 | 44 |
| Below $^{1}/_{2}$ of the average | 28 | 41 | 42 | 82 | 84 | 34 |

compared with two-fifths of Indian and Chinese households, and less than one-fifth of white and Caribbean households (Berthoud and Beishon, 1997). Caribbean households were more likely than others to contain one adult with children (i.e. were 'lone parent' households); about one in six Caribbean households had this structure, compared with less than one in twenty of others (Berthoud and Beishon, 1997).

Both the 1991 Census and the Fourth National Survey also provided detailed information on the socio-economic profiles of different ethnic minority groups. The following is a summary of key points from the Fourth National Survey (Modood et al., 1997), which are largely supported by data from the 1991 Census (Peach, 1996).

In terms of economic activity, the most striking findings concerned women. Eighty per cent of Bangladeshi and 70 per cent of Pakistani women described themselves as looking after the home or family, compared with about 30 per cent of white and Indian women, and only 13 per cent of Caribbean women. In contrast, most pre-retirement age men in all of the ethnic groups were in the labour market; differences here were largely due to different rates of unemployment, which were very high among Pakistani and Bangladeshi men (almost four times the white rate – see also Table 6.1) and also high among Caribbean men (more than twice the white rate). Detailed analyses showed that these higher rates of unemployment for Caribbean, Pakistani and Bangladeshi men persisted regardless of geographical location or qualifications, although the size of the differences varied (Modood, 1997a).

The Fourth National Survey included several indicators of socio-economic position. Again this is discussed in more detail in Chapter 6, but a summary indicator, equivalised household income, is shown in Table 1.3, which is drawn from Berthoud (1997). This shows the distribution of households according to average incomes and the great extent of poverty among Pakistani and Bangladeshi households. More than four-fifths of Pakistani and Bangladeshi households had below half the average income, a profile that is worse than that of white lone parents and white people post-retirement age (Berthoud, 1997). Two-fifths of Caribbean and Indian households were also in this position, compared with a third of Chinese and less than a third of white households.

Finally, no description of the lives of ethnic minority people in Britain would be complete without coverage of their experiences of racism. A central element of the Fourth National Survey was an attempt to assess the degree to which the lives of ethnic minority people were directly affected by racism. As part of this, white respondents were asked if they were prejudiced against certain ethnic minority groups. As many as one in five of the white respondents said that they were racially prejudiced against Caribbeans while one in four said that they were racially prejudiced against South Asians (in both cases slightly more for men and slightly less for women) (Virdee, 1997). In interpreting this figure, Virdee suggested that the crudeness of the question and under-reporting probably meant that this was an underestimate of the extent of racial prejudice among white people, but that the findings nevertheless indicated that 'a current of racist beliefs is clearly evident among a significant proportion of the white population' (Virdee, 1997: 278).

This was reflected in the widespread belief among the ethnic minority respondents to the Fourth National Survey that employers discriminated against ethnic minority applicants for jobs, and their reporting of widespread experience of such discrimination (Modood, 1997). There was also widespread experience of racial harassment reported in response to questions asking about being physically attacked, having property damaged, or being insulted for reasons to do with 'race' or colour. In response to these questions more than one in eight ethnic minority people reported having experienced some form of racial harassment in the past year (Virdee, 1997). Most of these incidents involved racial insults, many of the respondents reported repeated victimisation and a quarter of the ethnic minority respondents reported being fearful of racial harassment. The degree to which racial harassment is rooted in white British culture is indicated by the fact that the perpetrators of such incidents ranged from neighbours to people in shops, though they were predominantly strangers, and that the incidents occurred in almost all areas of the respondents' lives, including work. The fact that the racial harassment faced by ethnic minority people is part of their everyday interaction with white cultures was further emphasised by the finding that a significant number of those who had been harassed reported that the police were the perpetrators (Virdee, 1997).

## THE DATA USED TO EXPLORE ETHNIC DIFFERENCES IN HEALTH

As the introductory comments suggested, the epidemiological approach to work on ethnic health differences must be understood in the light of the type of data that have, to date, been available to researchers to explore the relevant issues. Consequently, before providing a brief review of existing literature on ethnic differences in health, this section will discuss the sources of data that have been used. The most influential work in Britain has been based on immigrant mortality statistics derived from national data sets. Country of birth is recorded on death certificates and has also been recorded in the decennial census, allowing an investigation of differences in mortality rates by both cause of death and country of birth (Marmot et al., 1984; Balarajan and Bulusu, 1990; Balarajan, 1996; Harding and Maxwell, 1997; Wild and McKeigue, 1997; Maxwell and Harding, 1998). However, despite the influence of these studies, there are several problems with data of this sort. Problems with the consistency of the recording of country of birth on death certificates and at the census means that it has been necessary to include fairly diverse groups in the same category, the most obvious of these being a category that includes all of those born in the Indian sub-continent (Marmot et al., 1984) – although Balarajan's (1996) and Harding and Maxwell's (1997) recent work attempts to improve on this situation. In addition to this, assessing ethnicity using country of birth is far from adequate, 'misclassifying' both ethnic minority people born in Britain and white people born overseas. For example, Peach and Winchester (1974) calculated that one-third of the people born in India and living in Britain at the time of the 1971 Census were white. And analysis of the country of birth and ethnicity questions at the 1991 Census show that at that time 15 per cent of those born in India described themselves as white and 88 per cent of these were aged 50 or more (Peach, 1996). In addition, it seems that there is a degree of inaccuracy in the recording of cause of death on death certificates (Cameron and McGoogan, 1981; Joint Committee of the Royal Colleges of Physicians and Pathologists, 1982). This inaccuracy in assigning cause of death has been shown to vary by occupational class (Bloor et al., 1989) and gender (Battle et al., 1987), so may well also vary by other characteristics of the deceased, such as ethnic background. This leads to the possibility that the recording of cause of death might be systematically biased by the influence of the ethnic background of the deceased on the recorder's decision making.

Also, if our concern is with the health of the population, mortality rates are a very crude indication of this complex multi-dimensional concept, an issue that is also discussed more fully in Chapter 2 in the section on measuring health. An equally important problem is that relying on census figures to determine the size of the 'at-risk' population can exaggerate the estimated risk for any group that is undercounted in the census, and, as has already been described, there is some evidence to suggest that such undercounting does vary by ethnicity as well as gender and age (OPCS, 1994). Finally, in terms of an epidemiological investigation that is concerned with exploring the aetiology of diseases that show variation, such data include no assessment of potential explanatory factors beyond occupational class as recorded at the census and on death certificates (potential problems with the use of these occupational class data for exploring ethnic inequalities in health are discussed in Chapter 6). Certainly there is no assessment of the often favoured biological and cultural explanations that are, as described earlier, consequently assumed, based on stereotypes and crudely used (Ahmad, 1993b).

In terms of other nationally representative data, general population surveys have not had sufficiently large samples of ethnic minority people for more than provisional conclusions to be drawn (see, for example, Benzeval et al., 1992), although this is changing as the Health Survey for England is expanded (Markowe, 1993; Erens et al., 2001). However, immigrant mortality data have been supplemented by smaller regional studies of the health of ethnic minority groups. Much of this work has had a general perspective (Pilgrim et al., 1993; Williams et al., 1993), but some has maintained an exclusive epidemiological focus on aetiology, where data from immigrant mortality studies are used to identify an ethnic group at greater risk from a particular disease, and then this greater risk is confirmed and aetiological factors explored in an in-depth local study. The work investigating the possibility that high rates of heart disease among South Asians are the result of an 'insulin resistance syndrome' is a good example of how this approach can be developed into a comprehensive research programme (McKeigue et al., 1988 and 1991; Cruickshank et al., 1991; Knight et al., 1992).

Despite the quality of much of this work, it still remains dependent on data that are far from adequate. Proportional mortality ratios are generally used for comparisons between ethnic groups by both local and national mortality studies that attempt to overcome crude ethnic classifications (Balarajan et al., 1984; McKeigue and Marmot, 1988). This is because the size of the population of different ethnic groups is unknown, and if the size of the population in which deaths are occurring is unknown, then the death rate for that population and a comparison with the general population (usually expressed as a standardised mortality rate) cannot be calculated. To overcome this the proportion of all deaths in the group due to a particular disease can be calculated, and that proportion can then be compared with that for the general population, giving a proportional mortality ratio. However, the limitations of proportional mortality ratios are well known (Roman et al., 1984). Particularly important is that they may not give a reliable estimate of comparative prevalence, because a high proportional mortality ratio for a particular disease can result from either a high relative prevalence of that disease or a low relative prevalence of other diseases. This means that such data require careful interpretation, particularly with regard to data on ethnicity, as immigrant mortality statistics suggest that death rates for some diseases in ethnic minority groups are relatively low (Marmot et al., 1984).

In addition, because of the highly concentrated geographical locations of particular ethnic groups in Britain (Owen, 1994a), described earlier, regional studies often cover only one specific ethnic group – such as Knight et al.'s (1992) study of insulin resistance and coronary heart disease among 'South Asian' men in Bradford, who were, presumably, predominantly Pakistani men, and McKeigue et al.'s (1988) study of coronary heart disease among Bangladeshi people in East London – but then have their results generalised to the wider population ('South Asian' in these examples) within which this group is included. Both the potential impact of factors associated with the specific ethnic group considered, and the locality within which that group is resident, are too easily ignored.

In terms of improving the data available for the study of ethnic differences in health, progress has been made over the last decade. First, for the first time the 1991 Census included a question on self-assigned ethnic group and another on the presence of a long-standing limiting illness. So far there has been little analysis of these data, although some is presented in Dunnell (1993), Owen (1994b, 1994c, 1994d and 1995) and Nazroo (1997a) and discussed later in this volume. Nevertheless, the Sample of Anonymised Records, which contains full Census data for 2 per cent of the population, allows for a detailed investigation of responses to the question on long-standing limiting illness. The main limitation of these data is their restriction to only one assessment of health, although the 2001 Census included a second question on self-assessed general health. This may be partly overcome by the routine and systematic collection of data on the ethnicity of patients admitted to hospital, introduced on 1 April 1996, which can be related back to population data derived from the census, although there may be some problems with this process (Aspinall, 1995). Additional problems with such data are that they only reflect the small hospital-treated proportion of those that are ill, a proportion that is likely to vary according to ethnicity (see the section on 'Mental illness' in this chapter and 'Measuring health' in Chapter 2). In addition, other factors of possible interest, such as socio-economic position, are not being collected alongside ethnicity in these administrative data.

Second, the Health Education Authority has carried out two surveys on the health and lifestyles of Black and minority ethnic groups (Rudat, 1994; Johnson et al., 2000). These studies have provided useful and unique information on a range of health behaviours, health promotion issues and health care, together with some on health status, for several ethnic minority groups in Britain. The main disadvantage with these surveys is that they were undertaken in areas with relatively large ethnic minority populations – those areas that, according to the 1981 Census, had 10 per cent or more of households headed by someone born in the Caribbean, South Asia or Africa – and, consequently, they were not fully representative of the populations they covered. Indeed, data presented by Smith (1996) suggest that such a strategy would cover only two-thirds of the ethnic minority population, and, of course, these two-thirds might differ from the remaining third in important respects. In addition, these surveys were unable to include a directly comparable general population group, and could only contain a limited coverage of other factors relevant to the lives of ethnic minority people. Nevertheless, they provide an important addition to our relatively limited knowledge of these issues.

Third, the Health Survey for England, the Department of Health's annual monitoring of the health of the population of England, has now included an ethnic minority 'boost' sample in its cycle of annual surveys. The first ethnic minority boost was conducted in 1999 (Erens et al., 2001), and contains unique data on the main ethnic minority groups in England (including Irish people). Importantly, this survey includes children, so it provides the only nationally representative data on the health of ethnic minority children currently available (Nazroo et al., 2001). This survey is medically focused, so concentrates on the measurement of disease – including 'objective' physical measurements – but unfortunately the focus on the measurement of disease means that there is little collection of explanatory data.

Fourth is the study reported here, the Fourth National Survey of Ethnic Minorities. The methods used in this survey will be described in full in Chapter 2; however, key points are: it is fully representative of the ethnic minority groups covered and includes a white comparison sample; health was assessed across a variety of dimensions, including both general health and specific illnesses; detailed information was collected on both ethnicity and features of the lives of ethnic minority people in Britain; and detailed information was also collected on demographic and socio-economic factors. This provides a rich and unique data source for examining the relationship between ethnicity and health. However, it does, inevitably, suffer from some disadvantages, two of which are worth mentioning here. First, its sample size was too small to explore the patterning of rare illnesses. In fact, the focus was almost exclusively on relatively common disorders (the exception being psychosis) that have been shown to vary by ethnic background. Second, it was based entirely on self-reported illness. No physical measurements were included, and it is possible that the relationship between self-report of illness and actual disease varied across ethnic groups, as it appears to do by class (Blane et al., 1996). A more detailed discussion of this issue can be found in Chapter 2.

## DIMENSIONS OF ETHNIC DIFFERENCES IN HEALTH

As described earlier, since the early 1970s ethnic differences in health have become an increasing focus of research in Britain. Summaries of current work can be found in: Balarajan and Soni Raleigh (1993 and 1995), who relate work on ethnic variations in health to the then Health of the Nation targets (Department of Health, 1992); Smaje (1995b), who provides the most recent comprehensive review of the existing state of affairs in research on health and ethnicity; Ahmad et al., (1996), an edited review covering three important dimensions of ethnic differences in health (cardiovascular disease, mental health and haemoglobinopathies); Ahmad (1993a) and Kelleher and Hillier (1996), both edited volumes that take a critical perspective on several of the key issues in this area; Marmot et al. (1984), a classic epidemiological study of immigrant mortality that has provided the model followed by many others; and Donovan (1984), whose critical review of the state of research up to the early 1980s shows that despite the exponential growth in the number of publications since his review, things have changed little since then. More recently there have been national surveys of variations in morbidity rates by ethnic group (Rudat, 1994; Nazroo, 1997a, 1997b; Johnson et al., 2000; Erens et al., 2001) and the tradition of analysing differences in mortality rates by country of birth has continued (e.g. Harding and Maxwell, 1997; Wild and McKeigue, 1997; Maxwell and Harding, 1998).

The following provides an overview of some of the key dimensions of ethnic differences in health, examining some of the key outcomes that have been considered for some ethnic groups in other large population-based studies and which form the focus of the empirical analysis in following chapters. These outcomes have been chosen to cover both general health and specific illnesses, and to reflect the range of different health experiences across different ethnic groups. As with the rest of this volume, the aim is not to provide a comprehensive coverage of all ethnic groups and every health outcome; rather it is to use certain examples to begin to develop principles that will aid our understanding of ethnic inequalities in health. This initial discussion will simply be a presentation of some of the key findings in the data, although, because of their contested nature, the data relating to mental illness will be discussed in more detail.

## General health

Differences in general health can be assessed using either responses to summary assessments of health or data on all-cause mortality. In terms of morbidity measures, preliminary analysis of the 1991 Census data, which for the first time included a question asking about long-standing illness that limits activities, suggested that the rate of such illness is greater among all of the ethnic minority groups compared with whites, apart from the Chinese (Dunnell, 1993). An analysis of the census question for the age group (16 and older) and areas (England and Wales) used to sample for the Fourth National Survey confirmed that Dunnell's conclusions applied to that population (Nazroo, 1997a). In contrast, analyses of the 1999 Health Survey for England (Erens et al., 2001) suggested that rates of limiting long-standing illness were not generally high in ethnic minority groups, with a high rate only present for the Pakistani and Bangladeshi groups; although in the 1999 Health Survey for England responses to the question covering self-assessed general health indicated poorer health for all of the ethnic minority groups covered, except the Chinese group, compared with the general population.

Analysis of the Health and Lifestyles national survey also suggested that ethnic minority people report poorer health than white people, with non-whites being almost 25 per cent more likely than whites to have said that their health was fair or poor, although ethnicity for this survey was assessed only through interviewers' observations (Benzeval et al., 1992). The Health Education Authority's survey of Black and minority ethnic groups suggested that differences were even larger, with rates of reporting fairly poor or very poor health being at least twice as high as those for whites in each of the ethnic minority groups covered (African Caribbean, Indian, Pakistani and Bangladeshi), although differences for questions asking about 'any illness' and limiting illness were smaller (Rudat, 1994). Regional studies in Bristol and Glasgow confirm the reports of poorer health among ethnic minority groups (Pilgrim et al., 1993; Williams et al., 1993). For example, the Bristol study reported that 50 per cent of its respondents described their health as fair or poor, compared to a general population figure that ranged from 16 to 37 per cent, depending on household income (Pilgrim et al., 1993).

Interestingly, these findings are not fully reflected in mortality rates. Immigrant mortality statistics have consistently shown that standardised all-cause mortality rates are only slightly higher among men and women born in the Indian sub-continent and women born in the Caribbean compared with the general population, and that they are lower for men born in the Caribbean (Marmot et al., 1984; Balarajan and Bulusu, 1990; Harding and Maxwell, 1997; Maxwell and Harding, 1998). In contrast, all-cause mortality rates for those born in Ireland and Scotland, but living in England or Wales, have been repeatedly shown to be substantially higher than those for the general population (Balarajan and Bulusu, 1990; Harding and Maxwell, 1997; Maxwell and Harding, 1998).

## Cardiovascular disease

Cardiovascular diseases are the physical health outcomes that have received the most attention from those interested in ethnic differences in health. They are also a major cause of ill-health, with around 40 per cent of deaths occurring in Britain being attributed to them. Marmot et al. (1984), Balarajan (1991), Harding and Maxwell (1997) and Maxwell and Harding (1998), using immigrant mortality data from 1970–78, 1979–83, and 1991–93 respectively, demonstrated large differences by country of birth in deaths attributed to cardiovascular disease.

The higher risk of heart disease for those born in the Indian sub-continent compared with others has been a consistent finding in these immigrant mortality data. For example, in the period 1970–72 the standardised mortality rate for those born in the Indian sub-continent aged 20–69 was 119 for men and 128 for women (Marmot et al., 1984), while in the period 1979–83 these had risen to 136 for men and 146 for women (Balarajan, 1991).[1] The later data also demonstrated that this excess mortality was particularly significant for younger age groups, with those aged between 20 and 40 having more than twice the national average mortality rate. In addition, Balarajan's (1991) comparison with Marmot et al.'s (1984) data suggested that this ethnic variation in coronary heart disease had not narrowed over time. This evidence is supported by both worldwide reports of higher rates of coronary heart disease among South Asians (McKeigue et al., 1989), and the greater prevalence of indicators of coronary heart disease morbidity (rather than mortality) among South Asians in Britain. For example, McKeigue (1993)

---

1    The differences between these two periods are slightly exaggerated by differences in the age profiles of particular ethnic groups in the population at these times.

demonstrated higher rates of abnormal ECG (electrocardiogram) changes in South Asian men, and hospital admissions for coronary heart disease also appear to be higher for South Asian people (Cruickshank et al., 1980; Fox and Shapiro, 1988).

In contrast to this, immigrant mortality data suggest that those born in the Caribbean, but particularly men, have lower rates of mortality from coronary heart disease than the general population (Marmot et al., 1984; Balarajan, 1991; Harding and Maxwell, 1997; Maxwell and Harding, 1998). For example, in the period 1979–83, Caribbean men had less than half the national average rate and Caribbean women had three-quarters of the national average rate (Balarajan, 1991).

These data have also consistently demonstrated that men and women born in the Caribbean were at much greater risk than others of dying from a stroke – during the period 1979–83 the figures were 76 per cent higher for men, and 110 per cent higher for women than for those born in Britain (Balarajan, 1991). The rates of mortality from a stroke were also consistently higher for those born in the Indian sub-continent when compared with those born in Britain – 53 per cent higher for men and 25 per cent higher for women during the period 1979–83 (Balarajan, 1991). One of the key risk factors for strokes is hypertension, and it also appears that those born in the Caribbean have much higher rates of hypertension than the general population. The rates of mortality from hypertensive disease were four times greater for men born in the Caribbean and seven times greater for women born in the Caribbean according to the data presented by Balarajan and Bulusu (1990), and Marmot et al., (1984) showed similarly high rates. Those born in the Indian sub-continent also appear to have higher rates of hypertension than the general population, though relative mortality rates from hypertensive disease are not as great as they are for those born in the Caribbean (Cruickshank et al., 1980; Marmot et al., 1984; Balarajan and Bulusu, 1990).

## Non-insulin dependent diabetes

Non-insulin dependent diabetes is an important cause of both morbidity and mortality. In addition, it is also considered to be a risk factor for a variety of other diseases, such as cardiovascular disease and renal failure. In fact, it has been suggested that insulin resistance, a syndrome leading to non-insulin dependent diabetes, may be responsible for the higher reported rates of coronary heart disease among those born in South Asia (McKeigue et al., 1989). The prevalence of diagnosed non-insulin dependent diabetes among South Asian people is reported to be over four times greater than that among the white population (Mather and Keen, 1985; Mather et al., 1987; Simmons et al., 1989; McKeigue et al., 1991; Erens et al., 2001). If undiagnosed diabetes is also considered, this may well be an underestimation of the true difference in prevalence (Simmons et al., 1989). Also, mortality directly associated with diabetes among those born in South Asia is two to three times that in the general population (Marmot et al., 1984; Balarajan and Bulusu, 1990). Those born in the Caribbean have a similar excess of mortality associated with diabetes (Marmot et al., 1984; Balarajan and Bulusu, 1990) and the prevalence of diagnosed diabetes among Caribbean people is thought to be at least twice the rate in the general population (Odugbesan et al., 1989; McKeigue et al., 1991; Erens et al., 2001). However, the relatively high rate of non-insulin dependent diabetes among Caribbean people has not, for them, been linked to an increased risk of coronary heart disease.

## Respiratory disease

Those born in both the Caribbean and the Indian sub-continent appear to have lower rates of mortality from respiratory diseases (bronchitis, emphysema, asthma and pneumonias), apart from tuberculosis, than the general population (Marmot et al., 1984; Balarajan and Bulusu, 1990; Harding and Maxwell, 1997). This appears to be particularly the case for chronic obstructive airways disease (bronchitis and emphysema). It has been suggested that this is a result of lower rates of smoking among the various ethnic minority groups (Marmot et al., 1984). However, mortality data are only available for those born in the Indian sub-continent as a combined group, and it has now been shown that some of the South Asian groups, particularly Bangladeshi people, have high rates of smoking (Rudat, 1994). Whether the high prevalence of smoking among particular South Asian groups translates into high rates of chronic obstructive airways disease for them is not known.

## Mental illness

The relative prevalence of mental illness among different ethnic groups in Britain is probably one of the most controversial issues in the health inequalities field. Given the topic, which potentially allows the alignment of mental disorder with ethnic minority status (Sashidharan, 1993), the controversial nature of the field is not surprising. And this controversy is aggravated by the complexity of conducting research on ethnic differences in mental illness and the consequent disputed nature of research findings. Much of this controversy has focused on the apparently high rates of schizophrenia and other forms of psychosis among the African Caribbean population. Evidence suggesting low rates of mental illness among the South Asian population, but high rates of suicide and attempted suicide among young South Asian women, has also caused controversy.

Although mental illness is a relatively common condition, it is difficult to measure and the defining characteristics are contested. Both the definition and the measurement of mental illness depend on the presence of clusters of psychological symptoms that indicate a degree of personal distress, or that lead to behaviours that cause such distress to others. The clusters of symptoms associated with particular forms of mental illness are clearly defined by psychiatrists (see, for example, WHO, 1992; American Psychiatric Association, 1995), although the elicitation of these symptoms for diagnostic or research purposes can be difficult, particularly in cross-cultural studies.

For current purposes it is useful to divide mental illness into two categories, psychotic and neurotic disorders. The former are less frequent, but result in more severe disability. They are thought to affect around one person in 250 (Meltzer et al., 1995) and typically involve a fundamental disruption of thought processes, where the individual suffers from a combination of distressing delusions and hallucinations. Delusions often involve some notion of being persecuted or that some external force is controlling the individual's thoughts, while hallucinations typically involve hearing voices talking about or to the individual.

Neurotic disorders are much more common than psychotic disorders. A recent national survey suggested that in the week before interview about one person in 16 was affected by such a disorder (Meltzer et al., 1995). They are usefully separated into two categories, anxiety and depression that, although common, do involve considerably more than a sense of anxiety or sadness. For example, an individual with clinically significant anxiety would experience severe physical symptoms of anxiety along with some restriction in his or her social activity as a result of the anxiety, while an individual with clinically significant depression would be sufficiently sad and distressed to lose interest in most things and to be brooding on things to such an extent that she or he could not concentrate and could not sleep properly.

## *African Caribbean people and psychosis*

Hospital-based research in Britain over the past three decades has consistently shown elevated rates of schizophrenia among African Caribbean people compared with the white population. African Caribbean people are typically reported to be three to five times more likely than whites (published figures range from 2.2 times to 13 times more likely) to be admitted to hospital with a first diagnosis of schizophrenia (Bagley, 1971; McGovern and Cope, 1987; Harrison et al., 1988; Littlewood and Lipsedge, 1988; Cochrane and Bal, 1989; van Os et al., 1996). These findings have been repeated in studies that have looked at first contact with all forms of treatment, rather than just hospital services (King et al., 1994), although the rates in one such study were only twice those of the white population (Bhugra et al., 1997). Some of the more recent of these studies have also looked at those of African ethnicity and have reported similarly raised rates of psychotic illness in this group (King et al., 1994; van Os et al., 1996). Explorations of the demographic characteristics of Black people admitted to hospital with a psychotic illness suggest that these illnesses are particularly common among young men (Cochrane and Bal, 1989), and some studies have suggested that the rates are very high among young African Caribbean people who were born in Britain – for example, Harrison et al., (1988) report that the rates of first contact with psychiatric services for psychotic illness among this group are 18 times the general population rate.

This evidence has, on the whole, been interpreted in one of two ways by commentators. Many have accepted these data as broadly valid and regarded them as an opportunity to investigate the aetiology of schizophrenia. From this epidemiological perspective, uncovering the reasons for the higher rate among African Caribbean people would help resolve issues regarding the causes of schizophrenia more generally (e.g. Glover, 1989; Sugarman and Craufurd, 1994). The kind of explanations considered for the higher rates of psychosis among African Caribbean people are similar to those that are considered for other ethnic inequalities in health in the epidemiological literature (outlined earlier in this chapter).

First, the different rates of schizophrenia could be a consequence of factors related to the process of migration. Social selection into a migrant group could have favoured those with a higher risk of developing schizophrenia, or the stresses associated with migration might have increased risks. There is evidence both to support and to counter these suggestions. Investigations of the rates of schizophrenia in Jamaica and Trinidad suggest that they are much lower than those for African Caribbean people in Britain and, in fact, similar to those of the white population of Britain (Hickling, 1991; Hickling and Rodgers-Johnson, 1995; Bhugra et al., 1996). This would suggest that the higher rates are either a consequence of factors related to the migration process, or of the circumstances surrounding the lives of ethnic minority people in Britain. However, if the higher rates were a consequence of migration, we would expect other migrant groups also to have higher rates. Evidence here is contradictory. On the whole, studies have suggested that other migrants to Britain, in particular South Asian people, do not have similarly raised rates (Cochrane and Bal 1989). But King et al., (1994) (see also Cole et al., 1995), in a unique prospective study of all ethnic groups coming into contact with health and social services in a region within London, found that the incidence rate for first onset schizophrenia was higher in all ethnic minority groups (including white minority groups) compared with the white British population. In addition, if the higher rates were a consequence of selection into a migrant group or the stresses associated with migration, one would expect the rates for those born in Britain to begin to approximate those of the white population. However, studies have suggested that rates of schizophrenia for African Caribbean people born in Britain are even higher than for those who migrated (McGovern and Cope, 1987; Harrison et al., 1988), suggesting that factors relating directly to the process of migration may not be involved, although these data (like most work in this area) are dependent on a very small number of identified cases.

As with all work on ethnicity and health, there has been discussion of the possibility that differences may be a consequence of some essential attribute of ethnicity, but little supporting evidence has been marshalled. So, beyond speculation, cultural factors have not been directly considered in research (for a good example of such speculation see Sugarman and Craufurd's (1994) discussion of the possibility that high rates of cannabis use among African Caribbean people might be an important explanatory factor for their apparently greater risk of schizophrenia). At the same time the evidence cited in the previous paragraph, which shows that there are important differences between African Caribbean people who stayed in Jamaica, those who migrated to Britain, and those who were born in Britain, suggests that the higher rates are not a straightforward consequence of differences in genetic risk. It has also been suggested that the rates of schizophrenia among African Caribbean people are at their greatest for the cohort born in the 1950s and 1960s, and that this may be a consequence of exposure to a particular prenatal hazard among women newly arrived in Britain, such as an infection unfamiliar to the mother's immune system (Glover, 1989). If this was the case, we should be able to identify a clear cohort effect in the prevalence of psychosis in the African Caribbean community, something that it was not possible to explore in previously available data.

The different rates might be a consequence of the discrimination and racism that ethnic minority people face in Britain. This could be a result of the actual process of discrimination and harassment, or a result of the social disadvantages that they lead to. The recent evidence on both the nature and extent of the harassment ethnic minority people are subjected to (Virdee, 1995, 1997) has already been discussed here, and it would not be surprising if the multiple victimisation to which some are subjected led to mental distress. It would also not be surprising if the poor, rundown, inner city environments and poor housing that many ethnic minority people live in, and their poorer employment prospects and standards of living (Modood et al., 1997), led to greater mental distress (King et al., 1994). As elsewhere in the ethnicity and health field (Sheldon and Parker, 1992), there has been considerable criticism of the failure to take into account explanatory variables related to social disadvantage in work that links ethnicity to poor mental health, as there is a strong possibility that these underlie the relationship (Sashidharan, 1993; Sashidharan and Francis, 1993). These authors suggest that ignoring the possibility that the relationship between ethnicity and health is a consequence of social disadvantage allows the theoretical alignment of psychiatric disorder with ethnicity; psychiatric disorder becomes one of the essentialised attributes of certain ethnic minority groups. And the suggestion that psychiatric disorder is a consequence of some inherent and stable characteristic of certain ethnic minority groups then leads to the culture and biological heritage of those groups becoming pathologised, supporting the racialisation process.

However, an approach that explained the higher rates of psychosis as a result of discrimination, harassment and other forms of social disadvantage would have to be reconciled with two pieces of evidence. First, evidence from the Fourth National Survey (Modood et al., 1997), discussed earlier (see Table 1.3), indicated that Pakistani and Bangladeshi people were the most disadvantaged ethnic minority groups, but they do not appear to have higher rates of any mental illness (Cochrane and Bal, 1989), although the evidence on their rates of mental illness is not conclusive. It is possible, however, that the particular and different ways in which ethnic minority groups are racialised could lead to different outcomes for different groups (Jenkins, 1986, provides an example of this in relation to employment). Second, it is also puzzling to note that rates of anxiety, depression and suicide are lower among African Caribbean people than among the general population (Cochrane and Bal, 1989; Gilliam et al., 1989; Soni Raleigh and Balarajan, 1992a and 1992b; Lloyd, 1993). (Although the most recent mortality data rates suggest that those born in the Caribbean have a similar rate of suicide to the general population (Soni Raleigh, 1996).) If greater exposure to various forms of social stress was the explanation for higher rates of psychosis, we would expect these more common outcomes of stress to be also more frequent in the African Caribbean population.

Despite the consistency of research findings showing that African Caribbean people have higher rates of psychosis, some commentators have not accepted the validity of these data and continue to suggest that a higher incidence remains unproven, arguing that there are serious methodological flaws with the research that has been carried out. (See Sashidharan, 1993, and Sashidharan and Francis, 1993, for comprehensive reviews of the problems with existing data.) In summary, these flaws particularly result from the reliance of most work on hospital admission data, which raises a number of linked problems:

- Until the 1991 Census, where a question on ethnic background was asked for the first time, there had been only limited and unreliable data on the size of the African Caribbean population from which hospital admissions are drawn, resulting in its possible underestimation and consequent overestimation of morbidity rates. It has also been suggested that this also may be a problem with estimates based on the 1991 Census, because ethnic minority people have been under-enumerated (OPCS, 1994). However, some have shown that even if the African Caribbean population was much larger than they had estimated, the rate of psychosis would still remain significantly greater than that in the white population (Harrison et al., 1988; King et al., 1994; van Os et al., 1996).
- It is also possible that the number of African Caribbean people admitted to hospital with a first ever episode of psychosis could be overestimated. Lipsedge (1993) suggests two ways in which this might happen. First, because of the differences in the ways that African Caribbean and white patients are treated by mental health services (as described below), African Caribbean patients may be more reluctant to disclose any previous psychiatric treatment. Second, high geographical mobility in this population might lead to records of previous admissions being missed. Both of these would result in studies of contact with psychiatric services

for psychosis overestimating the number of African Caribbean patients with a first admission.

- Given that not all of those with psychosis are admitted to hospital, it is also possible that the data reflect the differences in the pathways into care for different ethnic groups, which result in African Caribbean people being more likely than equivalent white people to be admitted. In support of this possibility there is a large body of evidence that suggests that African Caribbean and other Black people are over-represented among patients compulsorily detained in psychiatric hospitals, are more likely to have been in contact with the police or other forensic services prior to admission, and more likely to have been referred to these services by a stranger rather than by a relative or neighbour. This is despite their being both less likely than whites to display evidence of self-harm and no more likely to be aggressive to others prior to admission (Harrison et al., 1989; Rogers, 1990; McKenzie et al., 1995; Davies et al., 1996). (Bebbington et al., 1994, found that once diagnosis had been taken into account, ethnic background was not related to risk of compulsory admission to hospital, but, as the next point illustrates, psychiatrists' assessments of patients and consequent diagnosis might be influenced by the ethnicity of the patient.)

- It is also possible that differences in the attitudes of health care workers to different ethnic groups and difficulties in the diagnosis of schizophrenia may be involved. For example, McKenzie et al. (1995) showed that African Caribbean people with psychosis were less likely than equivalent whites to have received psychotherapy or antidepressants; Harrison et al. (1989) showed that although African Caribbean people were no more likely to have been aggressive at the time of admission, once admitted staff were more likely to perceive them as potentially dangerous both to themselves and to others; and Rogers (1990) showed that psychiatrists were more likely than police to consider African Caribbeans detained under Section 136 of the Mental Health Act as dangerous to others. Coupled with difficulties in diagnosis, these pieces of evidence suggest that the stereotypes that inform the behaviour of health care workers may make them more likely to diagnose African Caribbean people as psychotic.

- In addition, some have argued that the symptom profile for Caribbean schizophrenics is different from that for white schizophrenics and that they should be more accurately considered as having an atypical psychosis (Carpenter and Brockington, 1980; Littlewood and Lipsedge, 1981). However, both Harrison et al. (1988) and Harvey et al. (1990) showed that there were great similarities in the symptom profiles of Caribbean and white patients with psychoses.

Interestingly, very similar criticisms have been made of epidemiological work exploring ethnic differences in psychotic illness in the United States (Adebimpe, 1994). Taken together, these comments suggested that there are a variety of potential problems with existing work and, consequently, that there must remain some doubt about the higher rates of psychosis reported among the African Caribbean group. Indeed, although the study that is widely regarded as the strongest in this field (Harrison et al., 1988 and 1989) overcame a number of these problems – it adopted a prospective design that included all African Caribbean patients making first contact with both hospital- and community-based services, used a standardised clinical assessment to overcome potential biases in diagnosis, and used a similar general population survey as a comparison – it, inevitably, still contained significant methodological weaknesses that raised doubts about the validity of the conclusions drawn (Sashidharan and Francis, 1993). For example: the population denominators were indirectly estimated using 1981 Census data on country of birth of the head of household; the comparison group was not concurrent (they used the sample identified for Cooper et al., 1987) and, because it was identified on the basis of possible diagnosis while the African Caribbean group was identified by screening for ethnicity, there were important differences in case identification; and case identification was also dependent on identifying patients with first contact with psychiatric services, which has the problems described above.

## *South Asians, mental illness and culture-bound syndromes*

Rates of mental illness among South Asian populations appear, on balance, to be lower than those for the general population (Cochrane and Stopes-Roe, 1981; Cochrane and Bal, 1989; Gillian et al., 1989). However, these findings are not entirely consistent; some studies of overall psychiatric hospital admission rates suggest that South Asian people have similar rates of admission (Carpenter and Brockington, 1980; Dean et al., 1981). These lower rates also may not be consistent across type of disorder. Although rates of hospital admission for neurotic disorders are substantially lower than those for the general population (Cochrane and Bal, 1989), it seems that schizophrenia is as common, or possibly more common, among South Asian people than the general population, although not to the degree reported for African Caribbean people (Cochrane and Bal, 1989; King et al., 1994). Also, while rates of suicide among most groups born in the Indian sub-continent are equal to or lower than those of the general population, rates among young women are more than twice those of their white counterparts (Soni Raleigh and Balarajan, 1992a and 1992b; Soni Raleigh, 1996).

Given the types of social disadvantage faced by ethnic minority groups in Britain, the overall lower rates of mental illness among South Asian people are puzzling. It has been suggested that the lower rates could be a consequence of a protective Asian culture, which, in language that is reminiscent of the concept of social capital (though it predates its current popularity in the health inequalities field), it is argued, provides extended social support networks (Cochrane and Bal, 1989), although others have criticised the stereotyped basis of such conclusions (Sashidharan, 1993).

Indeed, in a small local survey in East London, MacCarthy and Craissati (1989) were able to show that levels of psychological distress were significantly greater for Bangladeshis compared with white respondents in similar situations. This led them to conclude that 'the hypothesis that the Bangladeshi group would experience less distress, or be more psychologically robust in the face of adversity was not confirmed' (MacCarthy and Craissati, 1989: 200).

It is possible that the differences between white and South Asian groups, and the inconsistencies in these, could, like those for the African Caribbean group, be a result of the methodological limitations of studies in this area. In addition to the difficulties of relying on treatment data, outlined above, the lower rates of mental illness among South Asian people could reflect language and communication difficulties, or a general reluctance among South Asian people to consult with doctors over mental health problems. More fundamentally, they may reflect a difference in the symptomatic experience of South Asian people with a mental illness compared with white people. In particular, it has been suggested that South Asian people may experience particular 'culture-bound' syndromes – that is, a cluster of symptoms that is restricted to a particular culture, such as sinking heart (Krause, 1989) – or may be more likely to somatise mental illness – that is, experience and describe psychological distress in terms of physical symptoms (Rack, 1982) – and consequently not be identified as mentally ill. For example, Williams et al. (1997) demonstrated that a standardised western assessment of psychological distress underestimated problems among South Asian people living in Glasgow relative to their white peers when compared with self-reported distress or a measure that more directly assessed somatic symptoms. And elsewhere Williams and Hunt (1997) showed that this under-estimation may have been specific to distress resulting from situations that were more commonly experienced by South Asian people, such as a low standard of living.

Kleinman (1987), in what comes close to a relativist perspective on mental illness, has suggested that the problems with cross-cultural psychiatric research may be even more fundamental. Somatisation is typically seen as a result of a different, culturally informed, mode of expressing the 'same' disorder – that is, a disorder with a similar biological basis. However, Kleinman (1987) suggests that the reliance on a biological definition of disease crucially undermines an understanding of how different the culturally shaped illness may be – differences in symptomatic expression reflect

> substantially different forms of illness behaviour with different symptoms, patterns of help-seeking behaviour, course and treatment responses ... the illness rather than the disease is the determining factor (Kleinman, 1987: 450).

Given the reliance of psychiatric research on the identification of clusters of symptoms that reflect an underlying disease and the potentially different idioms for mental distress used in different cultures, Kleinman (1987) argues that cross-cultural research can easily lead to what he calls a 'category fallacy'. The use for research or treatment in a particular culture of a category of illness that was developed in another cultural group may fail to identify many to whom it can apply, because it lacks coherence in that culture. The idioms of mental distress in the researched group are simply different from those used in the research tool. So Kleinman (1987) points out the obvious fallacy in attempting to identify the prevalence of 'semen loss' or 'soul loss' in white western groups. This may, of course, equally be the case for instruments designed to detect western expressions of neurotic disorders when applied to other, particularly in this case South Asian, cultures. Indeed, Jadhav (1996) has been able to describe the historical and regional development of 'western depression', leading him to suggest that this apparently universal disorder is culturally specific.

There has only been limited empirical work in this area so there is only limited evidence to support this position. In one example, Fenton and Sadiq-Sangster (1996) identified an expression of distress that they described, using their respondents' words, as 'thinking too much in my heart'. While they found that this correlated strongly with the expression of most of the standard western symptoms of depression, they were also able to show that some of these standard symptoms were not present (those relating to a loss of meaning in life and self-worth), suggesting that at least the form that the disease took was different. They also pointed out that 'thinking too much in my heart' was not only a symptom as such, but a core experience of the illness, raising the possibility that there were more fundamental differences between this illness and depression.

## South Asians, mental illness and suicide

In contradiction with the apparent lower overall relative rates of mental illness among South Asian people, analyses of immigrant mortality statistics show that mortality rates from suicide are higher for young women born in South Asia, and that this is particularly the case for very young women (aged 15 to 24), where the rate is two to three times the national average (Soni Raleigh et al., 1990; Soni Raleigh and Balarajan, 1992a and 1992b; Karmi et al., 1994). In contrast to the findings for young South Asian women, these studies also showed that men and older women (aged 35 or more) born in South Asia had lower rates of suicide. Analysis of the most recent data on immigrant mortality has been more detailed, because it could be coupled with the 1991 Census and this included a question on ethnicity as well as country of birth (Soni Raleigh, 1996). This confirmed the pattern just described, but was able to show that the high rates were restricted to those born in India and East Africa. Both men and women born in Pakistan and Bangladesh had lower mortality rates from suicide than the general population, while women born in India and East Africa had higher rates, and men born in India and East Africa had similar rates.

In the attempt to explain the high mortality rates of suicide among young women born in South Asia, research has explored the reasons given by those who have attempted suicide. Analysis of the hospital records of such people has focused on cultural explanations for attempted suicide and particularly on a notion of culture conflict, where the young woman is apparently in disagreement with her parents' or husband's traditional or religious expectations (e.g. Merrill and Owens, 1986; Biswas, 1990; Handy et al., 1991). Although these reports are largely speculative, those who have extrapolated from them in order to explain the high mortality rates from suicide among young South Asian women have accepted such conclusions, locating the causes of these high rates outside individuals' mental health and saying that such instances of self-harm are a consequence of family pressures and conflict. For example, Soni Raleigh and Balarajan state:

> Most immigrant Asian communities have maintained their cultural identity and traditions even after generations of overseas residence. This tradition incorporates a premium on academic and economic success, a stigma attached to failure, the overriding authority of elders (especially parents and in-laws) and expected unquestioning compliance from younger family members. Thus, interpersonal disputes particularly in relation to marriage and lifestyles, the pressures of economic competition with the loss of self-esteem associated with failure, and the anxiety attached to non-conformist behaviour have been cited as causes of self-harm among the young (male and female) ... These pressures are intensified in young Indian women, given their rigidly defined roles in Indian society. Submission and deference to males and elders, arranged marriages, the financial pressures imposed by dowries, and ensuing marital and family conflicts have been cited as contributory factors to suicide and attempted suicide in young Indian women in several of the studies reviewed here. (Soni Raleigh and Balarajan, 1992a: 367).

However, a closer examination shows that such stereotypes may not hold and there are, in fact, great similarities between the motives of white and South Asian patients for their suicidal actions. For example, Handy et al. (1991) say that arguments with parents were a common factor for both the white and Asian children in their study, and Merril and Owens' (1986) examples of 'restrictive Asian customs (e.g. not allowing them to go out at night, mix with boys, or take further education)' (p. 709) are not greatly different from what one might find in a dispute between a young white woman and her parents. Indeed, a study of coroners' reports in London found that only one-third of the twelve South Asian women who had committed suicide had 'family conflict' cited among the reasons for the suicide, and only by stretching the imagination could these be considered as specific to South Asian cultures (Karmi et al., 1994). As Lipsedge has pointed out, it is likely that what would be described as 'parent–child conflict' among white families is 'anthropologised' by medical staff as clashes over cultural values rather than as personal difficulties or the everyday dynamics of family life ... Thus culture itself becomes a form of pathogenesis (Lipsedge, 1993: 176).

## *Summary*

The review suggests that many basic questions concerning the relationship between ethnicity and mental health remain unanswered. There remains a question of whether the use of western psychiatric instruments for the cross-cultural measurement of psychiatric disorder is valid and produces a genuine reflection of the differences between different ethnic groups (Kleinman, 1987; Littlewood, 1992; Jadhav, 1996). This has been raised particularly in relation to the low detection and treatment rates for depressive disorders among South Asians, but may apply to other disorders and other ethnic minority groups. It is also likely that treatment-based statistics do not accurately reflect the health experiences of the populations from which those in treatment are drawn. Two recent general reviews of the literature on ethnicity and mental health have pointed to the need for better data in this area, and particularly data derived from general population or community surveys (Smaje, 1995b; Cochrane and Sashidharan, 1996). Finally, as others have pointed out (Sashidharan and Francis, 1993), to avoid essentialising ethnic differences in mental health, there is a need to explore the factors associated with ethnicity that may explain any relationship between ethnicity and mental health, such as the various forms of social disadvantage that ethnic minority people face.

## CONCLUSION

This introduction has pointed to the lack of clarity in empirical research on ethnic differences in health. The lack of clarity can be considered to be a consequence of the 'untheorised' nature of much of the empirical activity in this field, where the ontological status of an ethnic categorisation is addressed only by implication. It is evident that much of the work has essentialised ethnic categories, assuming that they reflect homogeneous racial or cultural entities and, as such, provide useful markers of genetic or behavioural risk. Indeed, some diseases that show clear ethnic variations in prevalence, such as haemoglobinopathies, are based on genetic factors that vary across ethnic groups. There are also research programmes investigating whether more common diseases – such as diabetes, Coronary Heart Disease (CHD) and hypertension – are influenced by genetic factors that vary across ethnic groups (Wild and McKeigue, 1997). However, where biological markers have been found for more common diseases – such as insulin resistance syndrome and waist-to-hip ratios – it is not clear whether these are a consequence of genetic differences or environmental effects. The issue is further confused by the possibility that these biological differences may not only be a consequence of current environmental effects, which are hard enough to assess; they could also be a consequence of lifetime cumulative environmental effects, childhood and prenatal environmental conditions, and the individual's mother's living environment (Barker, 1991). And for those diseases that appear to be genetically determined, such as the haemoglobinopathies, it is evident that although the underlying genetic patterns vary across ethnic groups they are not exclusive to particular ethnic groups. In addition, for such diseases, it is clear that the severity of the illness is largely determined by environmental factors. For example, among those with the sickle cell gene the severity of manifest symptoms appears to be at least partly related to current environmental factors, such as diet and housing, and many of the problems faced by those suffering from sickle cell anaemia are related to the inadequate care that is available to them, which, in turn, is related to the ways in which Black people are perceived in Britain (Anionwu, 1993; Davies et al., 1993; Hill, 1994; Atkin and Ahmad, 1996).

Of course, cultural differences might contribute to ethnic variations in health in a number of ways, but most importantly through influencing health-related behaviours. For example, patterns of smoking and drinking have been shown to vary across ethnic groups. However, as described earlier, in health research culture is typically mapped onto reified ethnic categories and essentialised (Ahmad, 1993b). It is important for health researchers to remember that culture is not static, and that health behaviours are influenced by other factors as well, such as gender and class. Ahmad sums up this position well:

> Stripped of its dynamic social, economic, gender and historical context, culture becomes a rigid and constraining concept which is seen somehow to mechanistically determine people's behaviours and actions rather than providing a flexible resource for living, for according meaning to what one feels, experiences and acts to change. Cultural norms provide guidelines for understanding and action, guidelines which are flexible and changing, open to different interpretations across people and across time, structured by gender, class, caste and other contexts, and which are modulated by previous experiences, relationships, resources and priorities. The rigid conception of culture, which all too often is apparent in health research, serves a different function, however, it provides a description of people which emphasises their 'cultural' difference and helps to obscure the similarities between broadly defined cultural groups and the diversity within a cultural group (Ahmad, 1996: 190).

So when considering cultural differences in health behaviours as an explanation for ethnic differences in health, there is a need to consider ethnicity in terms of social action – ethnicity as a hybrid identity (Hall, 1992; Modood, 1998) that is not just given, but which is also the target of social action, continually changed across contexts and over time and fused with elements from other cultures, and which exists alongside other competing and complementary identities (such as gender and class). Importantly, this active and anti-essentialist notion of ethnic identity emphasises the political process of ethnic affiliation at the expense of behavioural (including, of course, those behaviours relating to health) markers of ethnicity (Modood, 1998). And, of course, such ethnic affiliation could provide important symbolic and material resources that are health promoting.

Also important is that in his rejection of the post-modern in his anti-essentialist approach to ethnic identity, Modood (1998) describes ethnic groups as having 'collective agency' and that in identifying cultural groupings our 'most basic and helpful guide is not the idea of an essence, but the possibility of making historical connections, of being able to see change and resemblance' (Modood, 1998: 382). Central to this historical conception of ethnicity must, of course, lie an understanding of ethnicity as social relations, hence the need to consider the structural dimensions of ethnicity and how these might contribute to ethnic inequalities in health.

Here Miles's (1989) portrayal of racism as central to an understanding of ethnic or 'race' relations is of great use. When discussing the emergence of ethnic or 'race' categories (the 'ethnic moment') Miles writes:

> Potentially, the 'ethnic moment' may be mediated by racism because all racisms (irrespective of whether they are self- or other-referential) offer a specific reading of claims of collective origin, history and mode of being, one which signifies designated traits as a mark of nature. Thereby, the ethnic collectivity is reified as product of nature. Thus, all racisms entail, although in varying combination, the signification of a range of traits...in such a way as to collapse the analytical distinction between biology and culture (for which the ideas of 'race' and 'ethnicity' act as metaphors). The collectivity so designated is therefore made socially visible... This existential Otherness is not just portrayed as a 'fact' of difference, although this is a necessary moment. It is also a justification for differential treatment in the form of exclusion: racism is the preparatory moment of exclusion within the realm of ideological relations (Miles, 1996: 253).

In addition to the implicit critique of health research that adopts essentialist notions of ethnicity as culture or biology, this quote also reminds us that a core component of ethnic relations involves the categorisation of the Other and the exclusion of the Other. This points to potentially fruitful lines for investigating ethnic inequalities in health. At one level the experience of and recognition of racism and a devalued ethnic minority status might in itself have an effect on health through psychological mechanisms. For example, Benzeval et al. (1992) demonstrated that experiencing racial harassment was significantly associated with reported acute illness (after controlling for other relevant variables) and that experiencing any form of discrimination at work was significantly associated with both acute and long-standing illness. Also ethnic minority people have a clear recognition of the relative disadvantage they face and it is suggested that inequality in social position in itself can damage health, perhaps as a result of psychological processes that operate when social comparisons are made (Wilkinson, 1994 and 1996). There is growing evidence to support this possibility; for example, Ben-Shlomo et al. (1996) showed that the extent of *variation in income* in a location was related to increased mortality rates even after the relationship between average income in the location and mortality rates had been accounted for. It seems likely that the process of social comparison will be of more significance to the health of ethnic minority groups than the general population, as any social comparison made by ethnic minority people will clearly illustrate the obvious inequalities, discrimination, and racism, that they face in virtually all spheres of their lives (Modood et al., 1997). Indeed, recent evidence from the Fourth National Survey suggests that both the experience of racism and the perception of the operation of racist discrimination are adversely related to health (Karlsen and Nazroo, 2001a).

In addition, inequalities in access to health services have been well established in a number of studies. For example, although ethnic minority people are at least as likely as white people to consult with their GP, they are less likely than whites to leave the surgery with a follow-up appointment (Gilliam et al., 1989), or to receive follow-up services such as a district nurse (Badger et al., 1989). South Asian people with CHD wait longer for referral to specialist care than white people (Shaukat et al., 1993) despite appearing to be more likely to seek immediate care (Chaturvedi et al., 1997). And in one study they were less than half as likely to receive grafts for triple vessel CHD, despite having further progressed disease (Shaukat et al., 1997).

None of these studies has been able to explore reasons for these possible differences in quality of care. But elsewhere it has been shown that ethnic minority people are more likely than whites to find physical access to their GP difficult; have longer waiting times in the surgery; feel that the time their GP had spent with them was inadequate; and to be unhappy with the outcome of the consultation (Rudat, 1994). Part of this might be related to communication problems. In terms of language, a significant number of South Asian (particularly Bangladeshi women) and Chinese people find it difficult to communicate with their GP (Rudat, 1994; Nazroo, 1997a). And, as described earlier, there may be cultural differences in the expression of symptoms, making the use of western diagnostic approaches inappropriate for some groups, especially as far as mental illness is concerned. But whatever the exact mechanisms leading to ethnic inequalities in access to health services, part of the explanation may well be related to direct racist exclusion, and part to exclusion as a result of the geographical or class positions of ethnic minority groups.

The specific geographical locations of ethnic minority people might also make an important direct contribution to ethnic inequalities in health. There has been a great deal of research into the extent to which socio-economic inequalities in health are the result of the attributes of the areas where people live rather than the characteristics of individuals themselves (Townsend et al., 1988; Humphrey and Carr-Hill, 1991; Macintyre et al., 1993; Sloggett and Joshi, 1994; Gatrell, 1997). Aspects of the physical and social environment may influence both mental and physical health by influencing attitudes, structuring social interaction, limiting access to resources and increasing exposure to hazards (Robinson, 1989). For example, Macintyre et al. (1993) found that middle-class compared with working-class areas in Glasgow had easier access to, and cheaper, healthy food; more sporting and recreational facilities within easy reach; more extensive primary health services; and lower perceived crime risk.

The particular urban locations of the majority of ethnic minority people, which were described earlier, make them far more likely to have poor access to employment opportunities, good housing and other services, despite attempts to link resource allocation to patterns of deprivation (Robinson, 1989). These areas may also be more likely to be subjected to pollution and other environmental toxins that will have a detrimental impact on health. On the other hand, there is evidence to suggest that the concentration of ethnic minority groups in particular locations may be protective of health, allowing the development of a community with a strong ethnic identity that enhances social support, reduces the sense of alienation, increases the group's access to political power and protects against the direct effects of racism (Halpern, 1993; Smaje, 1995a; Halpern and Nazroo, 2000).

Finally, of course, central to this volume is the possibility that the class positions of ethnic minority groups make a major contribution to ethnic inequalities in health. To this end, once the methods to be used have been described, the following chapters will first describe ethnic differences in health using the necessarily crude ethnic classification available, then they will use additional indicators of ethnicity as identity/culture (religion and age on migration) to further explore ethnic differences in health, and finally go on to explore the contribution of socio-economic effects to ethnic inequalities in health. The conclusion will then, in the light of the empirical evidence presented in earlier chapters, revisit the discussion that has begun here.

# CHAPTER TWO

# Methods

## CONDUCT OF THE SURVEY

In 1993–94 the Policy Studies Institute, in partnership with Social and Community Planning Research (now the National Centre for Social Research), undertook a detailed survey of people from ethnic minority groups living in England and Wales – the Fourth National Survey of Ethnic Minorities (Modood et al., 1997). This built on the three earlier surveys carried out by the Policy Studies Institute and its predecessor, Political and Economic Planning, that charted the changing position of Britain's ethnic minorities from 1966 to the present day (Daniel, 1968; Smith, 1977; Brown, 1984). The survey was a national study covering England and Wales. It was based on a structured questionnaire that, in addition to health and health service use, covered many traditional measures of social and economic disadvantage, including sections on type and quality of housing, area of residence, employment, income, and education. In addition to this, several important issues were covered for the first time, including those relating to ethnic identity and the incidence and experience of racial violence and harassment. Findings from these sections of the survey can be found in Modood et al. (1997).

The survey was conducted in three phases.[1] First, a screening phase to identify the ethnic minority sample. Second, the main data collection phase, which covered both the identified ethnic minority sample and a white comparison sample. Interviewers were in most cases ethnically and language matched with respondents, and interviews were carried out in the language(s) of the respondent's choice. The languages used included: Urdu; Punjabi;

---

[1]    Full details of the survey methods, including copies of the materials used, can be found in the methodological report on this survey (Smith and Prior, 1997). Copies of the questionnaire used can also be found on the world-wide-web at:
http://kennedy.soc.survey.ac.uk/qb1/nav4/fr_home.htm.
The module containing the health questions can be found in Appendix A.

Gujarati; Bengali (Sylhethi); Hindi; and Cantonese. Translations of questionnaires and other materials were carried out by a commercial translation agency and were checked by having the translation independently translated back into English. These were then tested in three small-scale pilot studies and subsequently modified.

Third, given the difficulties with the cross-cultural assessment of mental health, outlined in Chapter 1, and the necessary reliance on a fully structured interview for the main stage of the Fourth National Survey, it was imperative to assess the validity of the mental health measures used. This led to the development of a follow-up study, also carried out by the Policy Studies Institute and Social and Community Planning Research, of those respondents whose answers suggested that they *possibly* had a mental illness. This involved such respondents undergoing a well-established detailed clinical interview undertaken by ethnically and language matched psychiatric nurses or doctors. Version 9 of the Present State Examination (PSE) (Wing et al., 1974) was chosen for the psychiatric assessment in this interview as it had already been translated into most of the languages required. The follow-up interview was also extended to provide coverage of treatment and use of health services. In many ways the design of this element of the study followed that of the OPCS National Psychiatric Morbidity Survey (Meltzer et al., 1995), although there were some important differences, which will be returned to later.

## SAMPLING

Great attention was placed on the sampling procedure to ensure that respondents recruited into the survey were fully representative of the communities from which they were drawn. The sampling procedures were designed to select probability samples of both individuals and households. The areas used for sampling were selected on the basis of data from the 1991 Census on the ethnic minority population size in enumeration districts and electoral wards. For the ethnic minority sample they included areas with few ethnic minority people, a population that has been ignored by other regional and national surveys of ethnic minority groups. This ensured that the wards and enumeration districts used represented those where less than 0.5 per cent of the population were members of ethnic minority groups (low concentration), those where between 0.5 and 10 per cent of the population were members of ethnic minority groups (medium concentration), and those where more than 10 per cent of the population were members of ethnic minority groups (high concentration). Once the sampling points were identified, the small user Postcode Address File was used as the sampling frame to identify households to be screened for inclusion in the study.

Screening for ethnic minority respondents was carried out in the field. In areas with a high ethnic minority concentration, suitable ethnic minority respondents were identified by asking at all of the selected addresses whether there was anyone living at the address who was of Caribbean, Asian, or Chinese origin. In areas with medium and low ethnic minority concentrations, screening was based on the principle of focused enumeration, a method that has been shown to provide good coverage of the targeted populations (Brown and Ritchie, 1981; Smith, 1996; Smith and Prior, 1997). This involves interviewers visiting every nth (e.g. 6th) address in a defined area and asking about the ethnic origin of those living at both the visited address and at the n–1 (e.g. 5) addresses on each side of the visited address. Consequently, non-visited addresses are asked about at two visited addresses. If a positive or uncertain identification is made at either of the visited addresses for the non-visited addresses, the interviewer then goes on to visit them in person.

In practice the detail of this procedure varied according to the ethnic minority concentration in the area to be covered. In areas of medium ethnic minority density, on the whole every sixth address along the street was designated for an initial visit, but in some areas with more concentrated ethnic minority populations every fourth address was so designated. In these cases, when interviewers were told that there were no eligible ethnic minority people living at the non-visited addresses they were permitted to record them as having been covered with no further visit being made. However, if at either of the relevant visited addresses the interviewer was told that one or more ethnic minority people lived at *any* of the intervening non-visited addresses, they were asked to make personal calls at *all* of the intervening addresses to try to ascertain the ethnic origin of the people living at them. In contrast to this, in areas of low ethnic minority density every tenth address was used for the focused enumeration process and, if during this process the interviewer was told at exactly which address an ethnic minority person lived, the interviewer was instructed to visit that address directly rather than to visit *all* of the intervening addresses. Any households identified in this way as containing one or more ethnic minority people were then used to obtain the ethnic minority sample. In order to maximise the efficiency of the sampling process, in households containing ethnic minority people two respondents were selected for interview whenever possible (if there were one or two eligible adults in the household, all were selected; if there were three or more eligible adults, two were selected at random).

To identify the white sample a more straightforward three-stage stratified design was used. First, a sample of wards was drawn. Second, from within each selected ward a sample of addresses were identified from the small user Postcode Address File. Finally, interviewers selected one random eligible adult (rather than a possible two, as in the case of ethnic minority households) from within each selected address. The sample of wards was drawn to include those that, according to the 1991 Census, had a concentration of ethnic minority households both above and below 0.5 per cent.

The final sample achieved at the main stage of the study consisted of 2867 white respondents (119 with Irish family origins and 94 with neither Irish nor British family origins) and 5196 respondents who were members of ethnic minority groups. If ethnicity is allocated according to family origins, of the 5196 ethnic minority respondents, 1205 were Caribbean, 1273 were Indian, 728 were African Asian, 1185 were Pakistani, 591 were Bangladeshi and 214 were Chinese. Other ethnic minority groups were not covered. The assignment of individuals into particular ethnic groups is, of course, a complex and controversial process. This will be discussed in detail later in the chapter.

Six weighting factors were applied to the data in order to deal with the complex sample design and to ensure that the survey sample represented the populations under study as closely as possible. These accounted for differences in the probability of selection into the study, variations in the response rate by ethnicity, age and gender, and differences in the age profile of the sample compared with the 1991 Census data.

The age and gender profile of the Fourth National Survey Sample is shown in Table 2.1. This illustrates the need for age and gender standardisation in order to make a comparison between the ethnic minority groups and whites. The white sample has a greater proportion of women than the African Asian, Pakistani and Bangladeshi samples. It also has a three times greater proportion of respondents aged between 65 and 74 and a seven times greater proportion of respondents aged 75 or over, compared with other ethnic groups. This is reflected in the mean age of the populations, which, when compared to others, is six years greater for white men and ten years greater for white women. Where appropriate, subsequent data will be presented once age and gender standardisation has been carried out (see Chapter 3 for a more detailed discussion of this). However, gender and age differences were looked for routinely in the data and where they were found they have been reported. Such a routine exploration does mean that a large

**Table 2.1    Age and gender profiles**

*Column percentages*

|  | White | Caribbean | Indian | African Asian | Pakistani | Bangladeshi | Chinese |
|---|---|---|---|---|---|---|---|
| **Gender** | | | | | | | |
| Male | 45 | 45 | 47 | 55 | 51 | 55 | 47 |
| Female | 55 | 55 | 53 | 44 | 49 | 45 | 53 |
| **Age** | | | | | | | |
| 16 to 34 | 34 | 53 | 48 | 48 | 56 | 55 | 54 |
| 35 to 64 | 47 | 41 | 45 | 49 | 41 | 42 | 42 |
| 65 to 74 | 12 | 5 | 5 | 3 | 2 | 2 | 3 |
| 75 plus | 7 | 1 | 2 | 1 | 1 | 1 | 1 |
| **Mean age in years (SD)** | | | | | | | |
| Men | 44 (18) | 40 (17) | 40 (16) | 37 (14) | 35 (15) | 37 (16) | 36 (13) |
| Women | 46 (18) | 37 (15) | 37 (16) | 36 (12) | 34 (13) | 33 (12) | 35 (15) |
| Total | 45 (18) | 38 (16) | 39 (16) | 37 (13) | 35 (14) | 35 (15) | 34 (14) |
| *Unweighted base* | *2867* | *1205* | *1273* | *728* | *1185* | *591* | *214* |

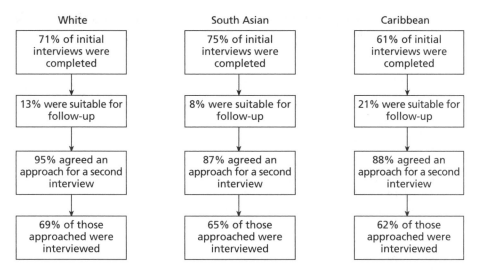

| White | South Asian | Caribbean |
|---|---|---|
| 71% of initial interviews were completed | 75% of initial interviews were completed | 61% of initial interviews were completed |
| 13% were suitable for follow-up | 8% were suitable for follow-up | 21% were suitable for follow-up |
| 95% agreed an approach for a second interview | 87% agreed an approach for a second interview | 88% agreed an approach for a second interview |
| 69% of those approached were interviewed | 65% of those approached were interviewed | 62% of those approached were interviewed |

**Figure 2.1    Response rates to the Fourth National Survey by broad ethnic group**

number of potential interactions between gender and ethnicity, and age and ethnicity, were explored, which, of course, raises the possibility that some of those reported were present in these data purely by chance.

## RESPONSE RATES

Response rates to both stages of the Fourth National Survey – the main stage and the follow-up validation stage – are shown in Figure 2.1 by broad ethnic group (South Asian groups are combined and the Chinese group was too small to be considered separately). Response rates to the main stage of the survey were comparable with those for the third Policy Studies Institute survey (Brown, 1984), and response rates to both parts of the survey were comparable with those reported for the National Psychiatric Morbidity Survey (Meltzer et al., 1995). In detail, among those who were approached for interview 71 per cent of white, 61 per cent of Caribbean, 74 per cent of Indian (including African Asian), 73 per cent of Pakistani, 83 per cent of Bangladeshi and 66 per cent of Chinese people agreed to take part. The lower response rate for Caribbean people at the main stage was the only ethnic difference of note here.

Because screening for the ethnic minority sample for the main stage interview was carried out in the field, some basic demographic information on some ethnic minority non-respondents could be collected.[2] This suggested that

---

2    The following discussion does not cover the Chinese group, which was too small to consider by age and gender, nor the white group, for whom there was no information collected on non-responders.

non-response was related to both age and gender. In terms of age, for all ethnic minority groups younger people were more likely not to have been interviewed. When comparing those aged under 35 with those aged 55 or more, the young compared with the old group were between about 15 per cent more likely, in the case of Bangladeshi and Caribbean people, to almost twice as likely, in the case of African Asian people, not to have been interviewed. Differences in response rate by gender were not so clear cut. For the Caribbean and Indian groups, men were more likely not to have been interviewed, for the African Asian and Pakistani groups there was no difference, and for the Bangladeshi group women were more likely to have not been interviewed. If both age and gender are considered, for all of the ethnic minority groups except Bangladeshi, young men were the most likely to be non-responders. Men aged under 35 compared with women aged over 55 were between about a third more likely, in the case of the Caribbean and Pakistani groups, to more than twice as likely, for the African Asian group, not to have been interviewed. For the Bangladeshi group, middle-aged men appeared to be the most likely sub-group not to be interviewed.

For the follow-up stage, response rates were similar for all groups. The lower overall response rate for the Caribbean group compared with the others is entirely a result of their lower rate at recruitment into the main stage interview. Figure 2.2 shows that the response rates for the follow-up for the interview for this study were not related to the reason for follow-up (the details of the follow-up criteria are described later).

Finally, of the 34 per cent of respondents for whom attempts to follow up had failed, around a third were the result of factors such as failing to make a second contact. Full details on this are shown in Table 2.2.

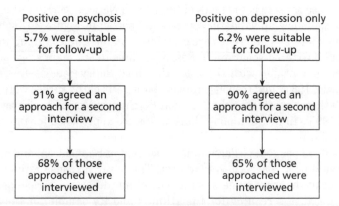

Figure 2.2   **Response rate to the follow-up interview by selection criteria**

**Table 2.2    Reasons for non-response at the follow-up stage**

|                                                        | Number | Per cent |
|--------------------------------------------------------|--------|----------|
| Addresses identified for follow-up                     | 845    | 100      |
| Unable to follow up (name of respondent missing etc.)  | 9      | 1        |
| Unproductive at interviewer visit:                     |        |          |
| Address empty                                          | 4      | *        |
| Moved, not retraced                                    | 32     | 4        |
| No contact                                            | 37     | 4        |
| Refused                                               | 85     | 10       |
| Other unproductive                                    | 19     | 2        |
| Appointment made for nurse/doctor visit               | 659    | 78       |
| Unproductive at nurse/doctor visit:                   |        |          |
| Refusal                                               | 39     | 5        |
| Broken appointment                                    | 37     | 4        |
| Other reason                                          | 28     | 3        |
| Productive nurse/doctor interview completed           | 555    | 66       |

\* less than 1 per cent.

## DEFINING ETHNIC GROUP MEMBERSHIP

As Senior and Bhopal (1994) point out, the concept of ethnicity is by no means simple. It contains notions of shared origins, culture and tradition and, as discussed in the introduction, involves anti-essentialist notions of identity and agency. So, in addition to recognising that ethnicity is a multi-dimensional concept, we need to acknowledge that it is neither stable nor pure, because culture is not an autonomous and static feature in an individual's life. It has a dynamic relationship to both the historical and contemporary experiences of social groups and the individuals within them (Ahmad, 1996). Central to the concept of ethnicity is that it is a reflection of the self-identification of individuals with particular cultural traditions. Certainly for members of ethnic minority groups there is an immediate and close link between self-identity and self-perceived ethnicity, although, as just suggested, self-perceived ethnicity and its link with identity is dependent on both immediate context and historical factors (Modood et al., 1994). In addition, there are competing claims on identity whose immediate relevance are also dependent on context, such as gender and class. The implication is that there are a range of (ethnic) identities that come into play at different times, and even, possibly, at the same time, and that (ethnic) identity should be regarded as neither coherent nor secure (Hall, 1992).

Despite the complexity of the concept of ethnicity, most research on health and ethnicity has taken a crude approach to the allocation of individuals into ethnic groups. As a recent *British Medical Journal* editorial pointed out, the categories of ethnic group used in health-related research are often undefined and inconsistently used (McKenzie and Crowcroft, 1994). This allows the status of ethnicity as an explanatory variable to be assumed, treated as though objectively measured and, consequently, reified. The view of ethnicity as a natural division between social groups allows the *description* of ethnic variations in health to become their *explanation* (Sheldon and Parker, 1992), leading, as suggested earlier, to untested assumptions about the existence and importance of cultural and biological differences being asserted as fact without underlying explanations being explored.

This has partly been a consequence of the limitations of available data. For example, as already discussed, because country of birth is recorded on death certificates and in the census, much of the published data in this area has allocated ethnicity according to country of birth, a strategy that is clearly inadequate. In addition, many studies use categories such as Black or South Asian to describe the ethnicity of those studied. Although some have suggested that this might be a useful starting point (Chaturvedi and McKeigue, 1994), it is important to recognise that such categories are heterogeneous, containing ethnic groups with different cultures, religions, migration histories, and geographical and socio-economic locations (Modood, 1994). In fact, rather than being a good starting point, combining ethnic groups is likely to lead to differences between them being ignored.

It seems that in order for work on ethnicity and health to progress further, assessments of ethnicity must be more adequate and the process used must be clearly defined (Senior and Bhopal, 1994). One way forward would be to acknowledge the dynamic and contextual nature of ethnicity, and to research the relationship between ethnicity and health with this explicitly in mind (Ahmad, 1995). However, such a task is difficult, if not impossible, to undertake in a cross-sectional quantitative survey, which inevitably must rely on a one-dimensional and relatively crude measure. Quantitative strategies require essentially arbitrary choices to be made about the appropriate demarcation of ethnic categories. An alternative to a truly contextualised assessment of ethnicity is to allow individuals to assign themselves into an ethnic group, which was the strategy adopted at the 1991 and 2001 Censuses. However, this suffers from a lack of stability; individuals often move themselves from one category to another when the question is repeated at a later date (Sheldon and Parker, 1992), a situation that is no doubt a reflection of the contextual nature of ethnic identity.

Another alternative, and the option used in the majority of the investigation presented in this thesis, is largely to ignore the role of self-perceived ethnicity and to assign ethnicity according to ethnic family origin. In this survey this was done by asking the question: 'Do you have family origins which are: Black Caribbean; Indian Caribbean; Pakistani; Bangladeshi; Indian; Chinese; Irish; white British; or did your family come from somewhere else?' Not surprisingly, perceived ethnicity and country of family origin are highly related, as Table 2.3 shows.

The approach based on country of family origin has the advantage of being a relatively straightforward and stable approach, although individuals within

## Table 2.3    Self-perceived ethnicity by ethnic family origins

*Column percentages*

| To which group do you belong? | White | Indian | African Asian | Pakistani | Bangladeshi | Caribbean | Chinese |
|---|---|---|---|---|---|---|---|
| White | 99.8 | 0.5 | 0.1 | 0.4 | 0.3 | 0.3 | 3.3 |
| Black Caribbean | 0 | 0 | 0 | 0 | 0 | 83.7 | 0 |
| Black African | 0 | 0 | 0 | 0 | 0 | 1.1 | 0 |
| Black Other | 0 | 0 | 0 | 0 | 0 | 0.3 | 0 |
| Black British | 0 | < 0.1 | 0 | 0 | 0 | 10 | 0 |
| Asian British | 0 | 0.8 | 0.8 | 0.6 | 0.3 | < 0.1 | 0 |
| Indian | 0 | 96.9 | 88.2 | 0.3 | 0 | < 0.1 | 0 |
| Pakistani | 0 | 0.6 | 6.0 | 98.3 | 0.2 | 0 | 0 |
| Bangladeshi | 0 | 0.2 | 1.0 | 0 | 98.8 | 0 | 0 |
| Chinese | 0 | 0 | 0 | 0 | 0 | 0 | 92.5 |
| Mixed | < 0.1 | 0.8 | 1.7 | 0 | 0.3 | 3.6 | 2.8 |
| Other | < 0.1 | 0.2 | 2.1 | 0 | 0 | 0.2 | 1.4 |
| Not answered | 0.1 | 0 | 0.1 | 0.4 | 0 | 0.7 | 0 |
| *Base* | *2867* | *1273* | *728* | *1185* | *591* | *1205* | *214* |

particular groups cannot be considered homogeneous in respect of a number of factors that may be related to both self-perceived ethnicity, such as religion or country of birth, and health, such as socio-economic status. Here it is particularly important to recognise that in this investigation the white group has been treated as though it reflects a homogeneous ethnic group, and one that has had its ethnicity left largely unquestioned. Some basic analyses of ethnic differences in mental health among the white group have been presented in Nazroo (1997b), but this is clearly an issue that needs to be tackled in future work (Sheldon and Parker, 1992; Bradby, 1995; Ahmad, 1999). Related to this, the most obvious practical problem with this approach is how to deal with respondents who identify themselves as having mixed family origins. Here, a crude approach of wherever possible allowing ethnic minority status to override white status has been taken. Again, as Table 2.4 shows, this has only affected a small number of respondents in the South Asian groups and less than 10 per cent of those in the Caribbean and Chinese groups.

Although the use of country of family origin to allocate ethnicity in this relatively crude and one-dimensional way is limited (see Ahmad and Sheldon, 1993, and Ahmad, 1999, for a discussion of the utility of such standardised measures of ethnicity and the relative costs and benefits of including them in surveys), it does enable a level of clarity to be maintained when making initial explorations of ethnic variations in health. And, importantly, it allows the exploration of this topic to move beyond the even cruder assessments of

**Table 2.4    Mixed ethnicity by ethnic family origins**

*Column percentages*

| | White | Indian | African Asian | Pakistani | Bangladeshi | Caribbean | Chinese |
|---|---|---|---|---|---|---|---|
| | | | **Ethnic family origins** | | | | |
| Responses to family origins and group membership questions suggest mixed ethnicity | 1.2 | 2.5 | 2.5 | 0.6 | 0.7 | 8.2 | 7.5 |
| *Base* | *2867* | *1273* | *728* | *1185* | *591* | *1205* | *214* |

ethnicity that are based on country/continent of birth, or over-arching categories such as Black or South Asian. The implications of using more sophisticated attempts to assign ethnicity in a survey such as this are explored in Chapters 4 and 5 of this book and returned to in the conclusion.

For the analysis that will be presented later, some ethnic groups have had to be combined in order to have sufficiently large sample sizes for robust estimates of difference. The way in which groups have been combined was designed to achieve a balance between sensitivity to differences between groups and the need for sufficiently large numbers of respondents with particular characteristics in each group. Throughout, the Indian group has been combined with the African Asian group, and the Pakistani group has been combined with the Bangladeshi group, as their responses followed very similar patterns. In some of the more detailed analysis it has been necessary to combine all four of the South Asian groups into one. Clearly such a combination leads to an unsatisfactory loss of detail about possible differences between South Asian groups. However, how the differences (and similarities) between these groups might influence the interpretation of data where they have been combined can be estimated from the findings presented elsewhere for individual groups (Nazroo, 1997a and 1997b).

In this volume the Chinese group has not been covered, because its small size would not permit the detailed analyses conducted here, and the very different health profile of Chinese people compared with all of the other ethnic minority groups meant that they could not be combined. Basic physical health findings for people in the Chinese group are reported in Nazroo, 1997a, while basic mental health findings for them are reported in Nazroo, 1997b.

## MEASURING HEALTH

Much of the work that has explored the social patterning of health has concentrated on mortality rates (e.g. Townsend and Davidson, 1982; Marmot et al., 1984). These have the advantages of being clearly defined, reasonably easily available from a combination of death certificate and census data, and reasonably disease-specific. However, in addition to the problems with the validity of mortality data that are described in Chapter 1, they are only a narrow reflection of what is clearly a complex concept. For example, the Health and Lifestyle Survey (Blaxter, 1990) showed the multi-dimensional nature of lay concepts of health, which included, among others, notions of 'not being ill'; not having, or overcoming, disease; a reserve or a source of energy; physical fitness or functional ability; and a sense of well-being. Certainly mortality rates reflect only a small element of these concepts. In addition, mortality rates may well not reflect even the narrowly defined disease-based definitions of health. The relationship between disease and death depends on a number of factors, including whether the disease is fatal, the types of treatment offered and used, and the wider resources available to individuals that affect the prognosis of a disease. Of particular importance to investigations of the social patterning of health is that such resources will vary across social groups. Given their differences, mortality and morbidity rates need not necessarily show the same social patterning.

In terms of asking questions about health in a survey such as this, with a focus on morbidity rather than mortality, a variety of strategies could be adopted. First, health can be considered in a medical sense as the absence or presence of recognised disease. For this, questions can ask directly about the presence of particular diseases, and this is one of the strategies adopted here. Data presented later will include responses to questions asking about the diagnosis of heart disease, hypertension and diabetes. However, such a strategy does raise certain problems, which partly result from how opportunities for the diagnosis of particular diseases might vary by social group. Certainly, a study of ethnic variations in health that relies solely on the identification of already diagnosed disease is particularly vulnerable to the criticism that differences in treatment rates and quality of treatment between ethnic groups, as well as differences in illness behaviour leading to differences in consultation rates and opportunities for diagnosis, may have produced the pattern of results reported. In addition to this, such questions are also dependent on the accuracy of respondents' knowledge and recollections of diagnoses that have been made. This will be influenced by the quality of the consultation with the doctor, which may also vary by social group.

Second, questions on disease can be extended beyond those on diagnosis to include coverage of symptoms. This helps to get around problems relating to differences in the access to or the use of medical services. Questions on symptoms were included in this survey, and will be reported later in relation to heart disease, respiratory disease, depression and psychosis (the last two of which are discussed in detail in the next section). However, such an approach cannot overcome possible differences between social groups in how these questions are interpreted and responded to. It seems possible that an assessment of whether a particular symptom is severe enough to be worth mentioning will vary across social groups, because of cultural differences in health beliefs, idioms for expressing symptoms, social roles and illness behaviour, particularly if the questions have been translated into different languages for different groups. Answers to such questions, consequently, may also produce misleading conclusions about differences between these groups.

A third approach is to ask about the effects of ill-health on the functioning of the respondent, although again the interpretation of such questions will be influenced by differences in social roles. For this survey the strategy adopted was to ask respondents to estimate the extent to which their performance of specific functions, such as climbing stairs, was restricted as a result of their poor health. A fourth possibility, also included here, is to ask respondents to provide a global self-assessment of their health. It has been suggested that the subjective nature of health makes this the most valid approach to assessing health (Benzeval et al., 1992), and there is some evidence that such self-assessments predict mortality rates (Mossey and Shapiro, 1982). However, like reports of symptoms, differences across social groups in both the reporting of functional limitation as a result of ill-health and the reporting of self-assessed health may be a result of differences in the way these groups interpreted the questions used.

This discussion of the four types of morbidity assessment used in this survey illustrates one fundamental difficulty with the interpretation of responses – in terms of making comparisons across ethnic groups, differences in responses may be a reflection of differences in the ways in which particular groups interpret and respond to questions and differences in their access to health care and the type of treatment received. Indeed, the problems faced here are similar to those discussed in some detail by Blane et al. (1996) in relation to assessing class differentials in morbidity, and McKinlay (1996) in relation to assessing gender differentials in health. Despite the difficulties with these assessments of health, some confidence in the responses to them in this survey can be taken from two pieces of evidence. First, *within* particular ethnic groups the social patterning of ill-health for all four modes of questioning was as would be expected, with the rate of ill-health being related to age, gender, smoking and socio-economic position. Second, where comparisons can be made between the four modes of questioning – for example, comparing responses to questions on diagnosis with those to questions on symptoms, or responses to questions on general health with those to questions on functional limitation as a result of ill-health – similar patterns of response *across* ethnic groups are shown for all but one question.[3] This suggests that on the whole all four types of questions on morbidity had some validity for exploring patterns of ill-health both within and across ethnic groups. In addition, the use of a 'battery of standardized instruments' in this survey increases the confidence with which we can interpret the findings (Blane et al., 1996).

---

3    The discrepancy involves responses to a question asking about 'long-standing illness', which others have suggested is interpreted differently by different ethnic groups (Pilgrim et al., 1993; Rudat, 1994), and which is explored at length in Chapter 3.

## CONTENT OF THE SURVEY

Much of the questioning on health used in the survey was derived from the Health Survey for England (White et al., 1993), which itself generally uses well-established and validated questions. As a result of the large amount of material that was covered in this survey, some of the questions on health were asked of only half of the sample. These are identified in the following list and in the text describing the results of the survey. In terms of the coverage of the interview, the health section tackled seven broad areas:[4]

1   General health status
   a   Self-assessed health, including general health, long-standing illness and disability.
   b   Activities limited by the respondent's health, using the physical functioning questions contained in the Medical Outcomes Study Short-Form Health Survey (SF 36) (Ware and Sherbourne, 1992). (Only asked of half the ethnic minority sample.)
2   Cardiovascular disease
   a   Diagnosis of coronary heart disease, hypertension and stroke.
   b   Symptoms of coronary heart disease, using the Rose Angina questionnaire (Rose and Blackburn, 1986).
3   Other specific physical health problems
   a   Diagnosis of diabetes.
   b   Respiratory symptoms, using questions derived from the Medical Research Council Respiratory questionnaire (MRC, 1982). (Only asked of half the ethnic minority sample.)
4   Perceived weight and health-related behaviours, such as smoking and drinking. (Only asked of half the ethnic minority sample.)
5   Accidents requiring hospital treatment, using questions derived from the 1989 General Household Survey (OPCS, 1991). (Only asked of half the ethnic minority sample.)
6   Use of health services including hospital services, general practice, dentists, home helps etc. (Some parts of which were only asked of half the ethnic minority sample.)
7   Mental health
   a   Tiredness and problems with sleep. (Only asked of half the ethnic minority sample.)
   b   Affective disorders, using questions derived from the CIS-R (Lewis et al., 1992). (Only asked of half the ethnic minority sample.)
   c   Psychotic disorders, using questions derived from the PSQ (Bebbington and Nayani, 1995).

---

4   The actual questions used can be found in Appendix A.

Not all of these items will be covered in this volume. The key outcomes covered will be: general health status (1) – all items except registered disability; cardiovascular disease (2); other specific health problems (3); smoking (4); mental health – affective disorders (7b) and psychotic disorders (7c).

As described earlier, the follow-up stage of the survey involved validating the mental health component of the survey, namely affective disorder (7b) and psychotic disorder (7c). The detail of this validation process and its outcomes are described next.

## THE ASSESSMENT OF MENTAL HEALTH IN THE SURVEY

### Main stage interview

The initial assessment of mental health used in the Fourth National Survey was based on structured questions. These were adapted from two instruments: the well-established revised version of the Clinical Interview Schedule (CIS-R) (Lewis et al., 1992) and the more recently developed Psychosis Screening Questionnaire (PSQ) (Bebbington and Nayani, 1995). The CIS-R is a standardised interview that covers neurotic disorders. It has been shown to be both a reliable and valid assessment of minor psychiatric disorder, and it has also undergone some cross-cultural validation (Lewis et al., 1992). It was designed for use by lay interviewers – it consists of structured questions with the respondents' replies taken at face value – so in this sense is ideal for use in a study such as the Fourth National Survey. The assessment of neurotic disorders in the CIS-R is based on 14 symptom groups: somatic symptoms; fatigue; concentration and forgetfulness; sleep problems; irritability; worry about physical health; depression; depressive ideas; worry; anxiety; phobias; panic; compulsions; and obsessions. This allows the CIS-R to be used as both an overall assessment of disorder and to generate diagnoses of specific psychiatric illnesses.

Although the CIS-R only takes 30 minutes on average to administer, this was far too long in the context of the Fourth National Survey. Two strategies were adopted to deal with this problem of length. First, only half of the ethnic minority respondents were asked the CIS-R schedule. Second, only certain of the 14 symptom groups it covers were considered. Focus was particularly placed on depression, and all of the questions for the depression and depressive ideas symptom groups (except a question on interest in sex) were asked. In addition, many of the questions on anxiety, phobias and panic, and the introductory questions in the sleep and fatigue sections, were asked. The most notable omission from the symptom groups covered was somatic symptoms. As discussed earlier, this may be especially important as far as South Asian respondents were concerned, because South Asian people may be more likely than others to experience and express mental illness in terms of physical symptoms.

The use of a standardised interview carried out by lay interviewers for the assessment of psychotic disorders is widely felt to be considerably more difficult than for the assessment of neurotic disorders. A set of standard questions is probably too restrictive to assess psychotic disorders, as a lack of insight into the disorder on the part of the respondent may produce misleading responses to the questions asked. The alternative of using a less structured approach to the assessment, with the interviewer making rating decisions, would require the interviewer to make clinical judgements and, consequently, she or he would need to have relevant clinical experience. For the main stage of the Fourth National Survey, which was restricted to the structured questionnaire approach, the PSQ was used. This was designed as a screening instrument that identified whether there was any possibility of the respondent suffering from a psychotic disorder. For example, in a recent assessment of its performance among a sample of psychiatric in-patients, psychiatric out-patients and GP attenders, only two out 124 respondents who screened negative on the PSQ were found to have a psychotic disorder when they underwent a full diagnostic interview (using the Schedules for Clinical Assessment in Neuropsychiatry – the SCAN) (Bebbington and Nayani, 1995). However, the use of such an instrument, while minimising the possibility of any false negative responses, does increase the false positive rate. The authors of the instrument suggest that if it is used in a population with a typical 1 per cent prevalence of psychotic disorder, for every six cases identified as positive by the PSQ only one would be a true case (Bebbington and Nayani, 1995). In order to reduce further the risk of false negatives, respondents to this survey were also asked about any medication they had used and any illnesses they had had diagnosed, so that those who had taken any anti-psychotic medication or had been given a diagnosis of psychosis could be identified and followed up.

## Validation of the main stage assessment

For a number of reasons neither the CIS-R nor the PSQ could be used in a straightforward diagnostic way. Although the CIS-R has been validated, only part of it was used here and it was not certain how the section used would perform on its own. Also, while there has been some cross-cultural validation of the CIS-R, because of language and cultural differences doubts remain about the effectiveness of such standardised assessments of neurotic disorder for cross-cultural research, particularly for South Asian populations. The PSQ has only been validated as a screening instrument, and its deliberately high false positive rate clearly means that there are important limitations to its use in a diagnostic sense. In addition it has not had any cross-cultural validation.

In order to assess the validity of these measures, respondents who met broad criteria suggestive of possible mental illness were approached for inclusion in a follow-up survey that, as described above, involved them undergoing a detailed well-established clinical interview based on version 9 of the Present State Examination (PSE) (Wing et al., 1974) and undertaken by ethnically matched psychiatric nurses or doctors. In an attempt to minimise the chances of missing any respondents who had a mental illness, the inclusion criteria used for the validation survey were as wide as possible. However, this does not mean that there were no false negatives and, as none of the respondents who were negative on all of the inclusion criteria were included in the follow-up, the full extent of this or whether it varied across ethnic groups cannot be assessed.

The detailed inclusion criteria for the follow-up study were:

8    From the CIS-R, any of the following answers:
   a    Yes to 'Have you felt unable to enjoy or take an interest in things during the past week?'
   b    Four days or more to 'Since last week on how many days have you felt depressed?'
   c    Yes to 'Have you felt depressed for more than three hours in total on any day in the past week?'
   d    No to 'In the past week when you felt depressed, did you ever become happier when something nice happened, or when you were in company?'
   e    Yes to 'Thinking about the past seven days, have you on at least one occasion felt guilty or blamed yourself when things went wrong and it hasn't been your fault?'.
   f    Yes to 'During the past week, have you been feeling that you are not as good as other people?'
   g    Yes to 'Have you felt hopeless at all during the past week, for instance about your future?'
   h    Yes to 'In the past week, have you felt that life isn't worth living?'
9    From the PSQ,[5] any of the following sets of answers:
   a    Yes to 'Over the past year, have there been times when you felt very happy indeed without a break for days on end?' and no to 'Was there an obvious reason for this?' and yes to 'Did your relatives or friends think it was strange or complain about it?'
   b    Yes to 'Over the past year, have you ever felt that your thoughts were directly interfered with or controlled by some outside force or person?' and yes to 'Did this come about in a way that many people would find hard to believe, for instance, through telepathy?'
   c    Yes to 'Over the past year, have there been times when you felt that something strange was going on?' and yes to 'Did you feel it was so strange that other people would find it very hard to believe?'

---

5    Those familiar with the PSQ will notice that one element, the question asking the respondent 'Have there been times you felt that a group of people was plotting to cause you serious harm or injury', was not included among the criteria for the follow-up. This question was felt to be too problematic for use among ethnic minority respondents.

    d   Yes to 'Over the past year, have there been times when you heard or saw things that other people couldn't?' and yes to 'Did you at any time hear voices saying quite a few words or sentences when there was no one around that might account for it?'

10  Reporting taking anti-psychotic medication or having a diagnosed psychotic disorder.

The follow-up interview allowed responses to the two sets of questions to be compared, so that the performance of the standardised questions in the main stage could be assessed and differences across ethnic minority groups could be analysed. This comparison will be the focus of the next section. However, before this is done, two of the limitations of the validation process are worth outlining.

First, the follow-up stage involved a fairly complicated procedure. Once the main stage interview had been undertaken, the coded data were entered onto a database. This was then immediately screened to see if the respondent met the follow-up criteria. The screening, therefore, was carried out on unchecked data and a small number of suitable follow-ups were missed and a small number of respondents were inappropriately followed up. If the respondent did meet the screening criteria, his/her name and address was then passed on to the follow-up study's field managers. They then arranged for the original interviewer to introduce to the respondent an ethnically matched psychiatric nurse or doctor, with appropriate language skills, who then carried out the follow-up interview. The demands of this process meant that there was a certain amount of time between the two interviews. The median gap was 17 weeks, and 80 per cent of the follow-up interviews were done between 9 and 26 weeks of the first interview. Even though interviewers for the follow-up study were asked to question about the period relating to the original interview, the distance in time between the two interviews clearly could have implications for the validation process, especially in terms of the accuracy of the recall of symptoms. However, there is no indication in the data that there was a relationship between the length of time between the interviews and the likelihood to meet the criteria for a PSE CATEGO syndrome (which are described in full later) in this sample.

Second, the validation process for the cross-cultural assessment of mental illness involved more than simply checking the performance of a crude assessment of psychiatric disorder with a more sophisticated one. As described earlier, all of the interviews were carried out in the language(s) of the respondent's choice. For the initial assessment using the PSQ and CIS-R, translations of the questionnaires and other materials were carried out by a commercial translation agency and were checked by having the translation independently translated back into English. For the PSE, if translations were already available they were used; where they were not bilingual, psychiatrists were asked to translate them. For this, back translations were not carried out, but the flexibility that the PSE allows a clinically trained interviewer should have minimised any problems resulting from inaccurate translation. Consequently, in so far as the validity of the measures depended on the accurate translation of *questions* into alternative languages, we can be reasonably confident, although this will be expanded on in more detail in Chapter 5.

However, as Kleinman (1987) has pointed out, the reduction of issues around translation to a purely technical problem of finding equivalent words or phrases ignores the possibility that the underlying concepts may differ across cultures. All of the instruments used in this research are clearly developed from within a western psychiatry model, so will inevitably fail to detect non-western culture-bound syndromes, or symptomatic expressions of disease that are differently determined by non-western cultures. The only safeguard the study had here was the use of ethnically matched interviewers. Given the flexibility allowed interviewers in the validation phase of the study, the degree to which the interviewer and respondent shared a culture may have enabled them to be sensitive to different culturally determined expressions of the same symptoms, even if different patterns of culturally determined symptoms for the same disease could not be identified. Even so, this may have been limited by the training in western psychiatry that all of the interviewers had undergone.

## Comparison with the National Psychiatric Morbidity Survey

At this point it is worth detailing the similarities and differences between the two elements of the Fourth National Survey and the National Psychiatric Morbidity Survey (Meltzer et al., 1995).

- Both the Fourth National Survey and the Psychiatric Morbidity Survey used the PSQ (which was, in fact, developed for the National Psychiatric Morbidity Survey) and the questions on diagnosis or treatment of a psychotic disorder. Both studies followed up respondents who scored positive on these questions, with one exception that is described next.
- An element of the PSQ – whether the respondent said yes to 'Have there been times you felt that a group of people was plotting to cause you serious harm or injury?' – was not included in the selection criteria for the follow-up to the Fourth National Survey, while it was for the National Psychiatric Morbidity Survey.
- While both studies also used the CIS-R, the Fourth National Survey used only part of it, with a particular focus on aspects relating to depression.
- Because of doubts concerning the effectiveness of western assessments of neurotic disorders among South Asian populations, the depression and depressive ideas elements of the CIS-R were part of the inclusion criteria for the follow-up validation interview in the Fourth National Survey. However, follow-ups in the National Psychiatric Morbidity Survey were carried out only on those who met one of the psychosis screening criteria.

- Finally, for clinical assessments in the follow-up element of the Fourth National Survey the PSE 9 was used together with additional sections on treatment and alcohol and drug use, while the National Psychiatric Morbidity Survey used the SCAN, which is constructed around the PSE 10.

## ASSESSMENT OF THE PERFORMANCE OF THE MENTAL HEALTH MEASURES

This section will be concerned with exploring the relationship between responses to the CIS-R and PSQ used in the initial fully structured main stage interview and responses to the PSE used in the follow-up clinical interview, and how this might vary across the ethnic groups included. It is important to remember that respondents who did not meet any of the CIS-R or PSQ criteria were not included in the follow-up. Consequently, little can be said about whether the initial questioning failed to identify some mentally ill respondents, and whether this varied by the ethnic origin of the respondents. As described earlier, both interviews were carried out by ethnically matched interviewers and in the language of the respondent's choice. However, the first interview was undertaken by 'lay' interviewers, whereas the second was undertaken by a psychiatric nurse or doctor who had received training in the use of the PSE.[6]

Table 2.5 shows the percentages of respondents who were suitable for follow-up according to each of the selection criteria (a respondent could, of course, meet more than one of the criteria). The data are age- and gender-standardised to allow for an immediate comparison of the ethnic groups.[7]

The most striking conclusion to be drawn from Table 2.5 is that those in both of the South Asian groups were less likely than those in the white group to be positive on both the CIS-R (depression) criteria and the PSQ (psychosis) criteria. In contrast, Caribbean people were slightly more likely than white people to be positive on the CIS-R criteria and were twice as likely to be positive on the PSQ criteria. The greater risk of Caribbean people to be positive on the PSQ criteria held for all of its components.

---

6  After the interviewers had been trained on the PSE, their performance was assessed by asking them to rate two taped interviews, one with a depressed patient and one with a schizophrenic patient. The result of this exercise was satisfactory. Ratings of the depressed patient for all interviewers produced a CATEGO class (essentially a diagnostic category, but see later for a description of this) of either neurotic or reactive depression. Ratings for just over three-quarters of the interviewers for the schizophrenic patient produced a CATEGO class of simple schizophrenia, one-fifth of the interviewers' ratings led to CATEGO class of depressive psychosis, and the remaining interviewer's ratings led to a class of non-schizophrenic psychosis.

7  These data do not show prevalence rates as only a proportion of those who screened positive actually turned out to be ill.

**Table 2.5    Respondents suitable for follow-up by selection criteria**

*Cell percentages: Age- and gender-standardised*

|  | White | Indian or African Asian | Pakistani or Bangladeshi | Caribbean |
|---|---|---|---|---|
| Positive on CIS-R (depression) criteria | 16.2 | 10.2 | 10.3 | 22.2 |
| *Unweighted base* | *2867* | *988* | *871* | *614* |
| Positive on any PSQ (psychosis) criteria | 5.5 | 3.3 | 2.5 | 10.8 |
| Hypomania | 0.4 | 0.2 | 0.1 | 0.7 |
| Thought insertion | 1.7 | 0.8 | 0.7 | 2.6 |
| Strange experiences | 3.6 | 2.7 | 1.7 | 7.5 |
| Hallucinations | 1.4 | 0.6 | 0.6 | 2.9 |
| Positive on psychotic medication or diagnosis criteria | 1.6 | 1.4 | 1.3 | 1.1 |
| *Unweighted base* | *2867* | *2001* | *1776* | *1205* |

When comparing the response rates to the follow-up shown in Figures 2.1 and 2.2, and the number of respondents suitable for follow-up shown in Table 2.5, with the number of respondents actually followed up, as shown in the following tables in this chapter, some additional points are worth considering. First, because only half of the ethnic minority sample were asked the CIS-R (depression) screening questions, in order to give white and ethnic minority respondents an equal chance of being followed up, only half of the white respondents who met the CIS-R criteria were approached for the follow-up interview. Second, because the process of selection for follow-up took place before the data had been fully checked, not all of the suitable respondents in Table 2.5 were correctly identified and approached, and some unsuitable respondents were followed up. Overall, 555 respondents were included in the follow-up and of these 24 did not meet the selection criteria. Those who did not meet the selection criteria are excluded from the following tables.

## The assessment of mental health at the follow-up stage

The PSE, which was used in the follow-up, involves the interviewer making an assessment of whether or not a series of 140 possible symptoms are present. If any symptom is judged to be present, an assessment is then made of its severity. The CATEGO computer programme[8] can then be used to derive

---

8    Here, rather than using the CATEGO programme, the symptom ratings from the PSE were entered into the SPSS-X statistical package. A programme was then written for SPSS-X that followed the CATEGO programme exactly and this was used to derive syndromes, categories, types and class.

syndromes, categories, types and eventually 50 hierarchical diagnostic classes. These 50 classes can be further reduced, using CATEGO criteria, to one of nine classes that include: schizophrenia; other schizotypal disorders; non-specific psychosis; psychotic depression; mania; depressive neurosis; and other neurosis. For the purposes of the validation exercise, the overall diagnostic process was considered in two stages.

First, the nine broad CATEGO classes were further combined to give three very broad hierarchical and mutually exclusive classes (described in descending order): a psychotic class (containing schizophrenia, other schizotypal disorders, and non-specific psychosis); a manic or psychotic depression class; and a neurotic class (containing depression, obsessional neurosis, anxiety and hysteria).

Second, the 38 syndromes, which the CATEGO programme directly derives from the symptoms rated by the interviewer, were combined in a direct way to reflect whether the respondent had any of the components of four broad symptom groups. These included syndromes suggestive of psychosis; neurotic depression; anxiety; and other neuroses. The detailed contents of each syndrome group were:

1   *Psychosis:* nuclear syndrome, catatonic syndrome, incoherent speech, residual syndrome, depressive delusions, hypomania, auditory hallucinations, delusions of persecution, delusions of reference, grandiose delusions, sexual and fantastic delusions, visual hallucinations, olfactory hallucinations, non-specific psychosis, depersonalisation and sub-cultural delusions.
2   *Neurotic depression:* simple depression, affective flattening, features of depression, self-neglect, worrying, ideas of reference, lack of energy, irritability, social unease, lack of interest/poor concentration, other symptoms of depression.
3   *Anxiety:* general anxiety and situational anxiety.
4   *Other neuroses:* obsessional neurosis, overactivity, slowness, agitation, tension, hypochondriasis and hysteria.

In contrast to the CATEGO classes, the CATEGO syndromes are a direct reflection of any and all symptoms reported by the respondent, so the programme naturally allows individuals to have more than one syndrome. This means that individuals are potentially counted in more than one syndrome group, but also means that none of the information on symptoms reported is lost, as it is in the hierarchical CATEGO class system.

Once the respondents in the follow-up study had been allocated into CATEGO classes and syndrome groups, comparisons could be drawn between the selection criteria for inclusion in the follow-up and responses to the PSE questions. The results of these comparisons are discussed next.

Table 2.6     Assigned CATEGO syndrome by criteria for inclusion in follow-up: all respondents

*Column percentages*

| | Selection criteria | | |
| --- | --- | --- | --- |
| | PSQ (psychosis) only | PSQ and CIS-R (depression) | CIS-R (depression) only |
| **Assigned CATEGO syndrome** | | | |
| Psychosis with or without neurosis[1] | 19    **20** | 23     **79** | 10 |
| Any neurosis, no psychosis | 47 | 67 | 66 |
| None | 34 | 10 | 24 |
| *Base* | *153* | *79* | *299* |

1 Very few respondents were assigned to a psychosis syndrome without neurosis, and the percentages here are reduced by less than 2 per cent in each column if those with only affective psychosis are excluded.

## Comparison of respondents' classifications at the first and second interviews

As described earlier, recruitment into the follow-up was based on the respondent meeting the criteria for possibly having either a psychotic illness or a neurotic depression illness or both. As a starting point to exploring how effective the screening instruments were for different ethnic groups, it is useful to see how the selection criteria into the follow-up were related to the final diagnostic ratings made. Table 2.6 does this by comparing the selection criteria with various combinations of CATEGO syndromes that the respondents were assigned to.

The table shows that a number of respondents did not meet the criteria for any CATEGO syndrome. However, given our aim to reduce the number of false negatives as far as possible in the selection process, at the risk of a number of false positives, this would be expected. One-fifth of those who had screened positive for psychosis were found to have a psychotic syndrome (the top cells of the first and second columns combined). Four-fifths of those who screened positive for neurosis were found to have a neurotic syndrome (the four cells in the top right corner of the table combined). Both these figures are much as would be expected given the screening accuracies built into the PSQ and CIS-R respectively. However, 10 per cent of those who only screened positive on CIS-R (depression) criteria were assigned a psychotic CATEGO syndrome (the top cell in the right hand column). This means that 30 out of the 73 respondents (41 per cent) who were assigned a psychotic CATEGO syndrome had not met the psychosis screening criteria. Similarly, 19 per cent of those who were assigned into a neurotic CATEGO syndrome were selected into the follow-up *only* on the basis of being positive on the psychosis screening. This raises the possibility that the screening was not as effective as had been hoped and that there were false negatives among the responses to the CIS-R and PSQ questions.

In order to explore the validation process further, the two selection criteria for the follow-up study will now be considered separately, although it is worth bearing in mind that 15 per cent of respondents were positive on both criteria.

## Validation findings for those positive on psychosis (PSQ) screening

Table 2.7 considers the CATEGO diagnostic class for respondents selected into the follow-up validation study on the basis of being positive on one or more of the PSQ (psychosis) items.[9] It shows a very similar pattern of response between the Caribbean and white groups, although slightly more Caribbeans were assigned a class of manic or depressive psychosis. The Indian or African Asian and Pakistani or Bangladeshi groups also had very similar patterns of response to each other. However, there were important differences between the two South Asian groups and the white and Caribbean groups. Although people in each of the ethnic groups were equally likely to be in a psychosis class, those in the two South Asian groups were less likely than others to be in a neurotic class and more likely to fail to meet the criteria for any class.

A check on these findings is provided by Table 2.8, which looks at the distribution of CATEGO syndromes for those positive on the PSQ screening. Whereas the hierarchical ordering of CATEGO classes meant that psychosis took priority over neurosis, this does not occur with CATEGO syndromes, where all of the symptoms rated by the interviewer are considered and respondents are potentially being counted in more than one group.

In fact, this table tells a very similar story to that told by Table 2.7. White and Caribbean people had a very similar distribution across the syndrome groups. The two South Asian groups also had a similar distribution to each other, but one that was again very different to that of the white and Caribbean groups. Despite having been just as likely to have a psychosis syndrome, South Asian people were less likely than white or Caribbean people to have any of the neurotic CATEGO syndromes and more likely to have no syndrome.

Overall, Tables 2.7 and 2.8 suggest that in terms of the main aim of PSQ screening, that is identifying those at risk of having a psychotic diagnosis or symptoms, the instrument gave a very similar result for all of the ethnic groups considered. Although overall only one in eight respondents met the criteria for a non-affective psychotic CATEGO class (one in six if affective psychosis is included and one in five if syndromes are considered), it is worth recalling that the PSQ was designed as a screening instrument that had as few false negatives as possible, even if that meant greatly elevating the number of false positives. In contrast, if neurotic CATEGO classes and syndromes are considered, differences between the ethnic groups appear. White and Caribbean people had similar patterns of response, with about

---

9    This does not include those respondents who reported taking anti-psychotic medication or a
     diagnosis of psychosis, but who did not meet the PSQ criteria.

**Table 2.7    Assigned CATEGO class for those positive on PSQ (psychosis) screening**

|  | | | | *Column percentages* |
|---|---|---|---|---|
|  | White | Indian or African Asian | Pakistani or Bangladeshi | Caribbean |
| Non-affective psychosis | 11.4 | 11.1 | 18.2 | 14.1 |
| Manic or depressive psychosis | 2.3 | 0.0 | 4.6 | 5.6 |
| Neurotic | 64.8 | 40.7[1] | 36.4[1] | 60.6 |
| None | 21.6 | 48.2[2] | 40.9 | 19.7 |
| *Base* | *88* | *27* | *22* | *71* |

1 p < 0.05 compared with the white group.
2 p < 0.01 compared with the white group.

three out of five meeting the criteria for a neurotic CATEGO class and only one-fifth having no CATEGO class, but people in both of the South Asian groups were less likely to be in a neurotic CATEGO class and more than two-fifths of them did not meet the criteria for any class.

# Validation findings for those positive on depression (CIS-R) screening

Tables 2.9 and 2.10 consider respondents who were included in the follow-up validation study on the basis of being positive on one of the CIS-R (depression) criteria. Table 2.9 gives the distributions for the hierarchical CATEGO classes for these respondents. Again, the white and Caribbean groups had a very similar distribution across the classes. However, those in the Pakistani or Bangladeshi group were considerably less likely than those in the white group

**Table 2.8    CATEGO syndromes for those positive on PSQ (psychosis) screening**

|  | | | | *Cell percentages* |
|---|---|---|---|---|
|  | White | Indian or African Asian | Pakistani or Bangladeshi | Caribbean |
| Psychosis | 20.5 | 14.8 | 22.7 | 22.5 |
| Depression | 75.0 | 51.9[1] | 50.0[1] | 73.2 |
| Anxiety | 44.3 | 18.5[1] | 13.6[1] | 40.9 |
| Other | 55.7 | 29.6 | 36.4 | 50.7 |
| None | 21.6 | 48.2[2] | 40.9 | 19.7 |
| *Base* | *88* | *27* | *22* | *71* |

1 p < 0.05 compared with the white group.
2 p < 0.01 compared with the white group.

**Table 2.9     Assigned CATEGO class for those positive on CIS-R (depression) screening**

| | | | | *Column percentages* |
|---|---|---|---|---|
| | White | Indian or African Asian | Pakistani or Bangladeshi | Caribbean |
| Non-affective psychosis | 7.5 | 10.6 | 8.5 | 9.5 |
| Manic or depressive psychosis | 2.7 | 3.0 | 2.1 | 0 |
| Neurotic | 72.9 | 62.1 | 44.7[1] | 73.0 |
| None | 17.0 | 24.2 | 44.7[1] | 17.6 |
| *Base* | *188* | *66* | *47* | *74* |

1 p < 0.01 compared with the white group.

to be assigned a neurotic CATEGO class and more likely to have no CATEGO class. Members of the Indian or African Asian group were also less likely than those in the white group to be assigned a neurotic CATEGO class, although this difference was not statistically significant.

Table 2.10 considers the CATEGO syndromes rated for respondents who had been positive on the CIS-R (depression) criteria. The similarity between the white and Caribbean profiles is again striking. As in Table 2.9, those in the Pakistani or Bangladeshi group were less likely than those in the white group to have any of the neurotic syndromes and this was reflected in their greater likelihood to be in the no syndrome group. Although those in the Indian or African Asian group were also less likely than white people to have an anxiety syndrome, differences here for depression were small and were not statistically significant.

The tables in this section suggest that the CIS-R operates in a similar way for the white and Caribbean groups. However, the finding in the previous section, that compared with white and Caribbean people, South Asian people

**Table 2.10     CATEGO syndromes for those positive on CIS-R (depression) screening**

| | | | | *Column percentages* |
|---|---|---|---|---|
| | White | Indian or African Asian | Pakistani or Bangladeshi | Caribbean |
| Psychosis | 14.9 | 13.6 | 8.5 | 9.5 |
| Depression | 79.8 | 72.7 | 51.1[1] | 77.0 |
| Anxiety | 48.9 | 13.6[1] | 19.2[1] | 39.2 |
| Other | 59.6 | 47.0 | 40.4 | 54.1 |
| None | 17.0 | 24.2 | 44.7[1] | 17.6 |
| *Base* | *188* | *66* | *47* | *74* |

1 p < 0.01 compared with the white group.

who screened positive for psychosis had lower rates of neurosis, is repeated for those in the South Asian groups who screened positive on depression criteria, although here significance tests suggest that the difference might be restricted to those in the Pakistani or Bangladeshi group.

## Summary

Tables 2.7 to 2.10 show a consistently similar pattern for the white and Caribbean groups. This suggests that the link between the measures used to assess mental health in the main stage and the follow-up interviews of the Fourth National Survey were equivalent for these two groups. Comparisons between the white and South Asian groups, however, showed a very different pattern. Although the match between the psychosis screening instrument and PSE rates of psychosis were similar for all of the groups, South Asian people were far less likely than either white or Caribbean people to meet the PSE criteria for a neurotic class or syndrome. This was particularly marked for those in the Pakistani or Bangladeshi group. Although it was also present for those in the Indian or African Asian group, there was a suggestion in Table 2.10 that this was largely a consequence of a lower rate of anxiety symptoms in the follow-up for this group.

The greater mismatch between CIS-R criteria and the PSE assessment for the South Asian groups compared with others can be explained in two ways. First, as suggested by the CIS-R results presented in Table 2.5, the South Asian groups may simply have had lower rates of neurotic disorders. This is supported by the suggestion in Table 2.5 that they also had lower rates of psychotic disorders, and by reports elsewhere of lower rates of psychiatric morbidity among South Asian people compared with the general population (e.g. Cochrane and Bal, 1989). If this was the case, the greater discrepancy between CIS-R and PSE assessments for South Asians could be explained as the CIS-R having a greater false positive rate for South Asians compared with others (in which case the figures for South Asians in Table 2.5 would be an *overestimate*). This would be consistent with our knowledge that the positive prediction value of a screening instrument decreases as the prevalence of the illness screened for decreases (Bebbington and Nayani, 1995). It is also possible that the time lag between the screening and validation in some way led to more in the South Asian groups than others recovering and forgetting their symptoms. This could be a result of their having less severe or shorter episodes of depression, perhaps as a result of their purported greater access to social support (Cochrane and Bal, 1989). However, as reported earlier, there is no evidence that the time lag between interviews did influence the reporting of PSE syndromes.

The second possibility is that both the CIS-R and the PSE were not adequate instruments for assessing neurotic disorders among South Asian populations. Such a possibility could explain both the apparently low prevalence of possible depression among the South Asian group according to the CIS-R screening criteria (Table 2.5), and the relatively low proportion of the South Asian groups who were positive on PSE neurosis criteria in both the CIS-R (depression) and PSQ (psychosis) parts of the follow-up validation survey (Tables 2.7 to 2.10). The possibility that both the CIS-R and the PSE assessments of neurosis did not perform well for South Asian groups is not entirely unexpected. As discussed in Chapter 1, when considering the measurement of subjective psychological phenomena it is important to recognise that the meaning of particular words and the concepts that underlie them could have great cultural variation (Kleinman, 1987). This could be a purely technical problem, which could be overcome by making sure that terms describing the appropriate concepts are adequately translated. In fact, for both the main stage and follow-up interviews for the Fourth National Survey, great care was placed on the translation of interviewer materials. In addition, care was taken to ensure that interviewers at both stages had the appropriate language skills and were ethnically matched, and, in the semi-structured follow-up interview, the interviewer had the flexibility to adjust the wording of questions if she or he deemed this appropriate. This should have meant that the technical translation difficulties involved in an inquiry about psychological phenomena had been minimised.

However, there are also the possibilities that the symptomatic expression of depression was different for those in the South Asian groups compared with members of the white group, or that in attempting to measure depression in this group we were committing what Kleinman (1987) has called a category fallacy (see Chapter 1 for a discussion of this). Indeed, the authors of the PSE appear to accept that it may be reflecting a particular culture when they state that

> the PSE incorporates the views of a school of thought which might reasonably be called Western European in its origins and which is shared by psychiatrists in many other parts of the world (Wing et al., 1974: 11).

If this is the case, then the assessments of depressive disorders among the South Asian groups in this study could be considered to be an underestimate of their true extent of mental disorder. This possibility is tested further in Chapter 5.

In contrast, the assessment of possible psychosis in the Fourth National Survey appears to have worked consistently across all ethnic groups, with a similar percentage of those positive on the PSQ screening criteria in each group meeting the PSE criteria for a psychotic diagnosis or syndrome. In terms of the anticipated performance of the PSQ, results are also much as expected. The one in eight of those positive on the PSQ who actually met the criteria for a diagnosis of a non-affective psychosis is consistent with the one in six that the authors of the instrument suggest is likely if it is used in a population with an overall prevalence of 1 per cent (Bebbington and Nayani, 1995). Interestingly, many of those who were positive on the PSQ criteria, but who did not meet the criteria for a psychotic CATEGO class, did meet the criteria for a neurotic CATEGO class.

The overall conclusions of the validation process appear to be that the PSQ (psychosis) indicators worked consistently across all ethnic groups. The CIS-R (depression) indicators worked consistently for the white and Caribbean groups, but did not work in the same way for the South Asian groups and may well have underestimated their rates of depression. The PSE similarly may have underestimated rates of depression in South Asian groups.

## ESTIMATING RATES OF MENTAL ILLNESS IN THE SURVEY SAMPLE

As described earlier, most, but not all, of the ethnic minority respondents who scored on the depression and psychosis parts of the initial interview underwent a follow-up clinical interview to assess their mental state more accurately. In the National Psychiatric Morbidity Survey (Meltzer et al., 1995) reasonably accurate assessments of affective disorder were made possible by the use of a standard algorithm to convert CIS-R scores into diagnostic categories. Here the use of a standard algorithm was not possible, because only a part of the CIS-R was asked of respondents. Nevertheless, as shown in Table 2.11, the greater the number of items that the respondents said 'yes' to on the depression and depressive ideas section of the CIS-R, the greater the likelihood that they met the criteria for a CATEGO class at the follow-up interview – only a quarter of those who scored on two or three items did not meet any CATEGO criteria and only one in twenty of those who scored on five or more items did not meet any of the criteria, and this relationship was statistically significant ($p < 0.001$, 9 d.f.).

More importantly, there was also a clear relationship between the CIS-R score and the likelihood of meeting the criteria for the neurotic depression class. Of those who scored one on the CIS-R, just under one in five met the criteria for neurotic depression compared to one in four for those who scored two or three; one in three for those who scored four; and one in two for those who scored five or more. However, because there was a significant number of respondents who did not meet the CATEGO criteria for neurotic depression despite scoring highly on the CIS-R, individuals could not be considered as cases or not cases on the basis of their CIS-R score alone. Instead the *likely* number of cases of neurotic depression within a particular population was estimated. This was done by using the relationship between the chance of meeting the criteria for neurotic depression and the number of CIS-R items scored – as shown in Table 2.11. That is, if a particular population had five people scoring on one item, five people scoring on two or three items, five people scoring on four items, and five people scoring on five or more items, the estimated weekly prevalence of neurotic depression would be: $(5 \times 0.17) + (5 \times 0.26) + (5 \times 0.36) + (5 \times 0.51) = 6.5$ people.

This, of course, assumes that the CIS-R and PSE worked uniformly across ethnic groups, which has earlier been shown not to be the case. If the relationship between CIS-R score and PSE class is considered for ethnic

**Table 2.11   Association between CIS-R scores and PSE CATEGO class (only those positive on CIS-R and followed up)**

*Column percentages*

| | CIS-R score on depression and depressive ideas and symptoms lasting more than two weeks | | | |
| | One | Two or three | Four | Five or more |
|---|---|---|---|---|
| **CATEGO class** | | | | |
| None | 37 | 26 | 10 | 5 |
| Other neurosis/anxiety | 37 | 44 | 40 | 23 |
| Neurotic depression | 17 | 26 | 36 | 51 |
| Psychosis | 9 | 5 | 14 | 21 |
| *Base* | *46* | *124* | *50* | *99* |

groups separately, the relationship is weaker for the South Asian groups. Despite this, for the estimated rates that are shown in the rest of this report it has been assumed that there was not an ethnic variation in the relationship between CIS-R scores and PSE classes. This has been done on the grounds that there were too few South Asians in the follow-up to produce accurate estimates for them alone, and that assuming no variation in confirmation rates by ethnic group would lead to a more conservative assessment of the differences between ethnic groups. Nevertheless it is worth bearing in mind that this has potentially led to an overestimate of the rates of neurotic depression in the South Asian groups – their rates would have been about 20 per cent lower if they were estimated using their lower confirmation rate.

In the standard use of the PSQ, respondents are not asked to continue the psychosis screening sequence once they have answered positively to one item. However, in the Fourth National Survey respondents were asked all of the questions regardless of their response to earlier ones. Consequently, a similar approach to that adopted for the CIS-R could be used to identify the risk of having a psychotic disorder. Table 2.12 shows the relationship between the number of items that respondents scored on the PSQ, or responses to questions on a diagnosis of psychosis or taking anti-psychotic medication, and the CATEGO class that they were allocated to at follow-up.

This shows a clear relationship between PSQ score and likelihood of meeting a psychotic CATEGO class, and this relationship was statistically significant (for all psychosis $p < 0.005$, 2 d.f., for non-affective psychosis $p < 0.02$, 2 d.f.). Consequently, the likely number of cases of psychotic disorder within a particular population was estimated in the same way as for the CIS-R and neurotic depression. This means that if a particular population had five people scoring on one item, five people scoring on two items, and five people scoring on three or more items or reporting a diagnosis of psychosis or taking psychotic medication, the estimated annual prevalence of non-affective psychosis would be: $(5 \times 0.09) + (5 \times 0.14) + (5 \times 0.22) = 2.25$ people.

**Table 2.12**   **Association between number of PSQ items scored and PSE CATEGO class (only those positive on psychosis screening and followed up)**

*Column percentages*

| | Number of PSQ items scored positive | | |
| | One | Two | Three or more or reports psychotic diagnosis/medication |
| --- | --- | --- | --- |
| **CATEGO class** | | | |
| None | 31 | 19 | 17 |
| Neurotic | 57 | 65 | 54 |
| Affective psychosis | 3 | 2 | 8 |
| Non-affective psychosis | 9 | 14 | 22 |
| *Base* | *143* | *43* | *65* |

This process is somewhat different to that used in the National Psychiatric Morbidity Survey (Meltzer et al., 1995), where only those who had been validated as a case in the follow-up PSE interview, or who had reported both taking anti-psychotic medication and having a psychotic illness, were considered as psychotic. Those who were not successfully followed up and who did not report both a diagnosis of and treatment for psychosis were excluded, a conservative approach that would inevitably lead to an underestimate of cases. As the National Psychiatric Morbidity Survey used the standard approach to asking the PSQ, where if the respondent scored on one question subsequent questions were not asked, the kind of estimates of the rates of psychosis made here could not be used. However, it is reassuring to note that if the National Psychiatric Morbidity Survey criteria are used for these data, an almost identical general population rate for non-affective psychosis is recorded. Less reassuring is that the estimate based on the strategy used here is about twice the 'official' estimate produced by the more conservative National Psychiatric Morbidity Survey criteria (the details of this are described later).

As for the estimated rate of neurotic depression, this process also assumes that the instruments used to assess psychosis performed uniformly across ethnic group. Tables 2.7 and 2.8 suggest that this was the case, but, because of the small number of respondents that were included in the follow-up on the basis of being positive on a psychosis item, it is impossible to be sure of this, or to estimate with any accuracy any variation in performance. However, a logistic regression model using the follow-up data suggests that the PSQ score was the only variable with a significant effect on predicting the outcome of being assigned a non-affective psychotic CATEGO class.

In addition to the assumptions outlined so far, the estimated rates of both neurotic depression and non-affective psychosis would be subject to sampling error. In this study sampling error would have occurred at both the main stage and the follow-up interview, making it extremely difficult to provide an accurate overall assessment of its effect. However, the degree to which sampling error might have affected the validation findings presented in Tables 2.11 and 2.12 is relatively straightforward to calculate, so this will be presented in the relevant tables as 95 per cent confidence limits (i.e. the range of values within which there is a 95 per cent probability that the true value lies), which can be found in brackets underneath the absolute rates. The small number of respondents followed up in both the CIS-R and PSQ parts of the sample make this range of values relatively large.

# CHAPTER THREE

# Ethnicity and health: patterns of disadvantage

## INTRODUCTION

As with almost all other research on the relationship between ethnic background and health, the primary focus of this chapter is to explore the extent of the difference between the health of the white and ethnic minority populations of England and Wales, rather than levels of ill-health *per se*. There are two potential reasons for adopting such a comparative approach. More commonly, as described earlier, a comparative approach is used within epidemiology in an attempt to explore the aetiology of particular disorders by identifying the groups at greater risk. Those groups who are at greater risk of the particular disease have, presumably, had greater exposure to certain aetiological factors that future research can set about identifying (see, for example, the rationale presented by Marmot et al., 1984, for undertaking their work on immigrant mortality rates). The limitations of such an approach have been discussed in Chapter 1 and will be returned to in the conclusion of this volume. A less common use of a comparative approach, though one fundamental to a critical enquiry, is to describe the health disadvantage faced by particular ethnic groups, to relate this to the other forms of disadvantage that they face, and to explore how disadvantage is structured by their minority status. This chapter provides a starting point to the latter process, by describing the relative chance of poor health across a variety of dimensions for three broad ethnic minority groupings compared with a white group.

However, while there is a clear importance in describing and attempting to explain inequalities in health across social groups, such an approach has the disadvantage of obscuring the actual health status of the groups concerned. A comparative analysis does not need to illustrate actual disease frequency, it only needs to demonstrate the rate of ill-health for a population that has been sampled and standardised to provide a valid comparison with other groups. Indeed, even standardised rates are often left out, with reports only containing a reference to odds ratios or relative risk. This means that actual rates of illness in communities and absolute greater risks between groups are hidden. An exclusive use of such a focus has several disadvantages.

First, health service planners need data that reflect absolute need rather than relative need if they are accurately to predict the services they should provide. Second, a focus on relative risk only allows assessment of changes over time in relation to the comparison group; assessment of changes within the group under study cannot be directly made. Third, a comparative analysis, particularly if it has an aetiological focus, will concentrate on those illnesses with a high relative risk for the population under study, which need not be those that contribute most to their burden of ill-health (Bhopal, 1997). Fourth, a comparison with a majority population often leads to the assumption that the majority population's experience is 'normal' and reasons for deviation from this should be found among the characteristics of the minority population(s), which are perceived to be deviant, and so opens up the possibility for racialisation. Finally, the use of gender- and age-standardised data obscures gender and age effects and the interactions between these and ethnicity.

For these reasons, it is important also to describe the actual health status of the groups we are covering. Consequently, the following tables contain unstandardised absolute per cent columns that represent the actual rates of reported illness in the ethnic group under consideration. And, to provide the comparative focus, the tables also contain an age-standardised relative risk column, with 95 per cent confidence intervals, for each of the ethnic minority groups. Relative risk is simply the chance of a member of one group to be in a particular category compared with a member of the other group. All of these comparisons were made with the white group. The confidence intervals give a range within which there is a 95 per cent probability that the true difference lies between the white and ethnic minority populations compared. Differences are statistically significant if the full range of values does not include the value 1. The age standardisation process will be described next.

## AGE AND GENDER STANDARDISATION

Given the large differences in the age profiles of ethnic minority compared with white groups (see Table 2.1), the relative risk data in this chapter have been age-standardised, and age- and gender-standardised where men and women are combined. This allows a straightforward comparison to be made between the health of the white group and the three ethnic minority groups. The standardisation process used here is direct standardisation, which involved using a weighting procedure to give each ethnic group the same age and, where relevant, gender structure. However, this procedure is dependent upon having relatively large numbers in each age and gender group used for calculating the weights, to prevent any amplification of a chance response. Unfortunately some ethnic groups had too small a sample size to be handled in this way. Consequently, those with Indian and African Asian family origins have been combined, and those with Pakistani and Bangladeshi family origins have been combined. Elsewhere, it has been shown that the groups that have been combined have very similar health profiles; the small differences between them can be seen in the relevant tables of Chapter 2 in Nazroo (1997a) and Chapter 3 in Nazroo (1997b). In order to allow the tables in this chapter to include the small number of elderly people in the minority groups, the standardisation process was done to the age structure of the total ethnic minority population. This means that only relative small weighting factors were applied to the few elderly ethnic minority respondents, reducing the chances of the weighting procedure biasing any result.

## SELF-ASSESSED GENERAL HEALTH

Several questions about general health were asked of all respondents. The first question considered here asked the respondent to rate his or her health on a five-point scale in relation to others of the same age (reported general health). Most reports dichotomise responses to this question between those who report 'excellent' or 'good' health and those who report 'fair', 'poor' or 'very poor' health, and the findings presented in Table 3.1 and Figure 3.1 are also based on this dichotomy.

Table 3.1 shows that members of the Pakistani or Bangladeshi group were overall about 50 per cent more likely than white people to have described their health as fair, poor, or very poor, and that this difference was similar for both men and women. Both men and women in the Caribbean group were also more likely than white men and women to have reported fair, poor, or very poor health. All of these differences are statistically significant. In contrast to the other ethnic minority groups, those in the Indian or African Asian group were very similar to the white group.

In terms of absolute rates, overall 32 per cent of ethnic minority people described their health as fair or poor. Not surprisingly, given the relative risks just described, the absolute per cent columns in Table 3.1 show that the rate for this was highest for those in the Caribbean and Pakistani or Bangladeshi groups. If just those who reported their health as poor or very poor are considered, 12 per cent of people in ethnic minority groups described their health in this way, and the figures were particularly high for the Bangladeshi or Pakistani group – around one in seven of these respondents described their health as poor or very poor.

Interestingly, all of the ethnic minority groups showed the expected gender difference, with women reporting higher rates of fair, poor, or very poor health than men, although differences were smaller for the South Asian groups. Of particular concern here is that very close to two-fifths of women in

**Table 3.1    Reported general health compared with others of the same age**

| | White | Indian or African Asian | | Pakistani or Bangladeshi | | Caribbean | |
|---|---|---|---|---|---|---|---|
| | Absolute % | Absolute % | Age-standardised relative risk | Absolute % | Age-standardised relative risk | Absolute % | Age-standardised relative risk |
| **Those reporting fair, poor or very poor health** | | | | | | | |
| Men | 26.2 | 25.9 | 1.06 (0.92-1.23) | 34.4 | 1.54 (1.35-1.76) | 32.8 | 1.26 (1.07-1.49) |
| Women | 32.0 | 29.8 | 1.01 (0.89-1.14) | 38.7 | 1.44 (1.29-1.61) | 39.1 | 1.31 (1.16-1.48) |
| Total | 29.4 | 27.8 | 1.03 (0.94-1.13) | 36.4 | 1.48 (1.36-1.61) | 36.2 | 1.29 (1.16-1.42) |
| *Unweighted base* | *2860* | *1996* | | *1771* | | *1201* | |

the Caribbean and Pakistani or Bangladeshi groups described their health as less than good.

Figure 3.1 shows how ethnic differences in reporting fair or poor health also varied by age. The higher rates among ethnic minority groups only began to emerge at the age of 35 and became greater (in absolute per cent terms) with increasing age. So, for the cohort aged 55 or older, all of the ethnic minority groups had much higher rates of fair, poor, or very poor health while, between the ages of 16 and 24, those in both the Pakistani or Bangladeshi group and the Indian or African Asian group had lower rates than white people, a difference that was statistically significant ($p < 0.01$) in both cases. Interestingly, this pattern is also present in data on social class inequalities in health, with class inequalities in health only emerging in older age groups, and it has been suggested that such findings are an 'artefact' resulting from the very low levels of poor health among the young (Blane et al., 1994).

Table 3.2 shows responses to questions asking respondents whether they have a long-standing illness and, if so, whether it limits their ability to carry out paid work. Considering any long-standing illness, which is similar to questions used in the General Household Survey and the 1991 Census (although it does not include the 'limiting' element of the equivalent census question), and absolute per cents first, overall one-fifth of the people in ethnic minority groups reported that they had a long-standing illness, although rates were much higher for the Caribbean than any other ethnic minority group.

In comparison with the white group, responses to the long-standing illness question suggest a very different pattern to that given in response to the reported general health question shown in Table 3.1. Rather than having

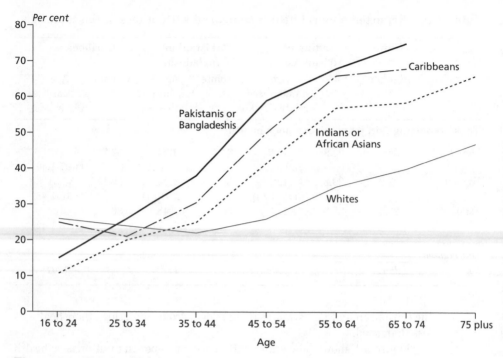

**Figure 3.1    Reported fair, poor or very poor health by age**

higher rates of long-standing illness than white people, those in the Caribbean group had similar rates and those in the Pakistani or Bangladeshi group had significantly lower rates. And, rather than having the same rate of long-standing illness as those in the white group, Indian or African Asian people had a rate that was less than two-thirds that of the white group. So, the two indicators of general health shown so far lead to opposite conclusions on ethnic inequalities in health.

Elsewhere there has been a suggestion that ethnic minority people interpret the long-standing illness question more restrictively than white people. A survey of ethnic minority people living in Bristol (Pilgrim et al., 1993) reported that its ethnic minority sample was less likely than the predominantly white sample in the Health and Lifestyles Survey (which it used for comparative purposes) to report a long-standing illness, a similar result to that shown in the first part of Table 3.2. However, many of the Bristol respondents who did not report a long-standing illness did report having one of a fairly exhaustive list of specific illnesses used in that study. This implies that the long-standing illness question was not an accurate reflection of existing illness, at least as far as ethnic minority respondents were concerned. The authors suggested that ethnic minority people may be less likely than white people to report an illness as long-standing because they have a more restrictive notion of what is serious enough to be included:

**Table 3.2    Reported long-standing illness**

| | White | Indian or African Asian | | Pakistani or Bangladeshi | | Caribbean | |
|---|---|---|---|---|---|---|---|
| | Absolute % | Absolute % | Age-standardised relative risk | Absolute % | Age-standardised relative risk | Absolute % | Age-standardised relative risk |
| **Any long-standing illness** | | | | | | | |
| Men | 31.8 | 16.6 | 0.61 (0.51-0.72) | 20.3 | 0.82 (0.70-0.95) | 30.0 | 0.90 (0.76-1.08) |
| Women | 33.6 | 17.4 | 0.64 (0.55-0.75) | 18.7 | 0.78 (0.67-0.91) | 30.1 | 1.11 (0.96-1.27) |
| Total | 32.8 | 17.0 | 0.62 (0.55-0.70) | 19.5 | 0.80 (0.71-0.89) | 28.7 | 1.00 (0.90-1.12) |
| **Long-standing illness that limits work** | | | | | | | |
| Men | 15.1 | 10.4 | 0.87 (0.68-1.10) | 14.4 | 1.33 (1.07-1.64) | 12.0 | 0.86 (0.64-1.16) |
| Women | 16.0 | 11.1 | 1.03 (0.82-1.30) | 9.6 | 1.06 (0.84-1.35) | 16.2 | 1.55 (1.24-1.94) |
| Total | 15.6 | 10.7 | 0.94 (0.80-1.10) | 12.1 | 1.20 (1.02-1.40) | 14.3 | 1.19 (0.99-1.42) |
| *Unweighted base* | *2865* | *1999* | | *1774* | | *1203* | |

It is possible that, in the case of Black and minority ethnic group respondents, the difference in response to a check list and to a general question is greater than for others ... It appears that people from Black and minority groups have a narrower interpretation of 'long-standing illness'. One explanation might be that 'long-standing illness' is interpreted as a condition which substantially and obviously affects daily living. Thus conditions such as asthma and diabetes are excluded (Pilgrim et al., 1993: 36).

This possibility is strengthened by Howlett et al.'s (1992) finding that Caribbean and white respondents to the Health and Lifestyles Survey favoured describing their health in terms of strength and fitness, while Asian respondents were more likely to favour describing their health in terms of being able to perform everyday activities. Interestingly, Rudat (1994) also reported difficulties with a long-standing illness question in the BMEG survey, and altered the wording in an attempt to overcome them.

In the data from the Fourth National Survey, a direct comparison between a comprehensive list of illnesses and reports of long-standing illness cannot be made, because no such list was used independently of the long-standing illness question. However, respondents were asked directly about diabetes, hypertension, cardiac disease and symptoms, and respiratory symptoms. For all of these except diabetes, ethnic minority respondents were no more likely than white respondents to say that they had the condition or symptoms while not reporting a long-standing illness. However, those in the South Asian groups were more likely than white people to say that they had diabetes while not reporting a long-standing illness. Of those South Asian respondents reporting diabetes, as many as 26 per cent did not report that they had a long-standing illness compared with just 12 per cent for the white group and 10 per cent for the Caribbean group (p < 0.01 for the South Asian group compared with the other groups combined).

The follow-up question asked of those who reported a long-standing illness – whether the long-standing illness limited the respondent's ability to work – also helps to resolve the contrasting patterns discussed so far. Responses to this can be found in the second half of Table 3.2, which shows a pattern quite contradictory to the less restrictive notion of a 'long-standing illness'. As with reported general health (shown in Table 3.1), those in the Pakistani or Bangladeshi group were significantly more likely than those in the white group to have reported a long-standing illness that limits the ability to work, the difference between the Caribbean and white group was close to statistical significance, and those in the Indian or African Asian group had the same rate as white people. This, together with the differences just reported for diabetes, suggests that the conclusions drawn by Pilgrim et al. (1993), on the differing interpretations across ethnic groups of the long-standing illness question, are correct.

A direct comparison between the questions so far used to assess general health also provides useful information on their validity for exploring ethnic differences in health. Within both categories of response to the long-standing illness question (i.e. those reporting and those not reporting a long-standing illness) ethnic minority respondents in all groups were more likely than white respondents to report that they had fair, poor, or very poor health, suggesting that for similar 'scores' on the long-standing illness questions, ethnic minority people had worse health than white people. Also, among those who reported good health, South Asian respondents were less likely than white and Caribbean respondents to report that they had a long-standing illness. These findings reinforce the belief that, compared with the other ethnic groups, South Asian people have to reach a higher threshold before they report a long-standing illness. Whether this overall pattern is a result of 'under-reporting' on the part of South Asian people or 'over-reporting' on the part of white people is not clear from these data, which suggest a combination of both explanations. For example, as just described, among those with diabetes South Asian people seem to 'under-report' the presence of a long-standing illness. However, among those reporting good health, white people appear to 'over-report' the presence of a long-standing illness.

In comparison with the reported general health question, the gender differences in reported long-standing illness, and long-standing illness that limits work, were also interesting. For those in the white and Indian or African Asian groups, women had slightly higher rates than men of both long-standing illness and long-standing illness that limits work, while for those in the Caribbean group women had similar rates to men of long-standing illness and higher rates of long-standing illness that limits work. In contrast, for the Pakistani or Bangladeshi group, women had lower rates of long-standing illness and markedly lower rates of long-standing illness that limits work. The contrast between this and the very clear pattern of gender inequality in response to the reported general health question (shown in Table 3.1) may be a reflection of the possible variations in the interpretation of these questions by different ethnic groups, as suggested above.

In fact, this pattern of findings has implications for the interpretation of the overall differences in self-assessed general health between ethnic minority groups. While, overall, the pattern among ethnic minority groups for long-standing illness that limits work was similar to that for any long-standing illness, with those in the Caribbean group having the highest rate and those in the Indian or African Asian group reporting the lowest rate, this overall pattern is, in fact, only approximately true when men and women are considered separately. Pakistani and Bangladeshi men had the highest age-standardised rates of long-standing illness that limits work and Indian or African Asian and Caribbean men had the lowest rates. In contrast, for women, those in the Caribbean group had the highest age-standardised rates of long-standing illness that limits work, while women in the other groups had remarkably similar rates. One interpretation of this is that the pattern of response to the second element of the long-standing illness question – whether it limits work – is at least partly dependent on patterns of paid working. Caribbean women have relatively high participation in paid employment, while Pakistani and Bangladeshi women have relatively low participation (Modood, 1997a), which may have led to an elevation in the numbers of Caribbean women who said that their illness limited work and a decrease in the numbers of Pakistani and Bangladeshi women who said this.

In order to get a more contextualised assessment of health, half of the respondents were asked if their abilities to perform a range of activities were limited by their health, using a sub-set of questions from the SF36 (Ware and Sherbourne, 1992). Responses to four of the specific activities asked about – the performance of moderate activities; climbing one flight of stairs; walking half a mile or more; and carrying groceries – were combined to provide an overall assessment of whether the respondent's health limited his or her ability to perform any of a range of moderately exerting activities. The findings for this are shown in Table 3.3.

In terms of absolute per cents, as many as 19 per cent of women and 12 per cent of men in ethnic minority groups had their performance of moderately exerting activities limited by their health. The table shows that this gender difference is consistent across all of the ethnic groups, although it was largest for the Caribbean group and smallest for the Indian or African Asian group.

Table 3.3   Activities limited by health

| | White | Indian or African Asian | | Pakistani or Bangladeshi | | Caribbean | |
|---|---|---|---|---|---|---|---|
| | Absolute % | Absolute % | Age-standardised relative risk | Absolute % | Age-standardised relative risk | Absolute % | Age-standardised relative risk |
| **Any of:** moderate activities; climbing one flight of stairs; walking half a mile; or carrying groceries | | | | | | | |
| Men | 11.8 | 12.5 | 1.59 (1.16-2.18) | 17.2 | 2.57 (1.95-3.37) | 8.3 | 0.83 (0.50-1.36) |
| Women | 22.2 | 14.8 | 1.08 (0.84-1.37) | 23.5 | 2.03 (1.67-2.48) | 21.5 | 1.54 (1.21-1.96) |
| Total | 17.6 | 13.7 | 1.27 (1.05-1.54) | 20.2 | 2.24 (1.91-2.63) | 15.5 | 1.29 (1.02-1.61) |
| *Unweighted base* | *2867* | *988* | | *873* | | *614* | |

Of the ethnic minority groups, overall those in the Pakistani or Bangladeshi group had the highest rate, one in five of them reporting that their health limited their performance of moderately exerting activities. However, among women, the difference between the Pakistani or Bangladeshi group and the Caribbean group was small, while Caribbean men were better off than other ethnic minority men.

Compared with the white group, members of each of the ethnic minority groups were significantly more likely to report one or more moderately exerting activity limited by health, with the rate being about 30 per cent more likely for the Caribbean and Indian or African Asian group and more than twice as likely for the Pakistani or Bangladeshi group. This is broadly consistent with the pattern of results for reported health (Table 3.1), and long-standing illness that limits work (Table 3.2). But responses to the questions on activities limited by health also showed important gender differences. Caribbean men had a very similar risk to white men of having one or more moderately exerting activities limited by health, while Caribbean women had a much greater risk than white women for this. For those in the Indian or African Asian group the pattern is exactly the opposite; Indian or African Asian women had the same rate as white women and men had higher rates than white men. There was no great gender variation in relative risk for the Pakistani or Bangladeshi group.

## Summary

These results for a range of indicators of general health illustrate the great burden of ill-health among ethnic minority people living in England and Wales. As many as a third reported that they had fair, poor, or very poor health, one-fifth that they had a long-standing illness and almost one in six that their performance of moderately exerting activities was limited by their health. However, the pattern of response was not uniform among the different ethnic minority groups. Those in the Caribbean and Pakistani or Bangladeshi groups reported the worst health across these three dimensions, while members of the Indian or African Asian group reported better health. Responses also varied across gender, with women on the whole reporting worse health than men for all of the ethnic minority groups, a pattern that was particularly striking for the Caribbean group.

Most of the assessments of general health used here lead to the conclusion that members of the Pakistani or Bangladeshi group had considerably worse health than white people. Caribbean people also had significantly worse health than white people, although for two of the indicators used this was the result of particularly poor health among Caribbean women. Those in the Indian or African Asian group had similar health to white people, although for one of the indicators Indian or African Asian men had a significantly higher rate of ill-health than white men. Differences between the ethnic minority and white groups also appeared to emerge only from the age of 35 and became striking around the age of 45, after which members of all of the ethnic minority groups were more likely to have had poorer health than those in the white group. However, this could be a result of the very low rate of reported general ill-health among the young obscuring ethnic differences at earlier ages (Blane et al., 1994).

Responses to the question asking respondents if they have a long-standing illness did not follow the pattern of response for other general health questions, with all ethnic minority respondents being less likely than white respondents to have such an illness. However, as others have shown (Pilgrim et al., 1993), there is some evidence to suggest that the long-standing illness question is not valid for making comparisons across ethnic groups, with some indication that white people 'over-report' and South Asian people 'under-report' such illness (e.g. white people reporting good health were more likely than others to report that they had a long-standing illness, while South Asian people with diabetes or reporting fair, poor, or very poor health were less likely than others to report a long-standing illness).

For these findings there is only one other national dataset with which comparisons can be made: the 1991 Census question asking about a limiting long-standing illness. During the development of the census question considerable work was put into assessing its reliability and validity (Thomas and Purdon, 1994). Although these assessments have not been reported by the ethnicity of respondents, responses to a follow-up interview during piloting do suggest that it is highly reliable. Of those reported as having a limiting long-standing illness on the census form, 88 per cent had this confirmed at the follow-up interview, while for those not reported as having a limiting long-standing illness, only 4 per cent were reported to have such an illness at the follow-up interview. In terms of validity, it was concluded that the 1991 Census question 'functions empirically as a (rough and imperfect) measure of disability' (Thomas and Purdon 1994: 10). Ethnic differences in this for the population from which the Fourth National Survey was drawn (white, Bangladeshi, Caribbean, Indian and Pakistani people aged 16 or older) were similar to the overall pattern for self-assessed general health that has been presented here. Compared with white people, Caribbean and Indian people had a relative risk of about 1.25 and Pakistani and Bangladeshi people had a relative risk of about 1.45 of reporting a limiting long-standing illness at the 1991 Census (see Nazroo, 1997a, for full details). If the census question is a valid indicator of health among white people, as the census reliability and validity assessment suggests, this would imply that among the Fourth National Survey questions it is the 'any long-standing illness' item that is most misleading, and that the other indicators of general health, which follow a similar pattern to both the census question and each other, should be regarded as the most valid indicators of ethnic differences. This supports the conclusions drawn earlier.

## CARDIOVASCULAR DISEASE

### Heart disease

Respondents were asked several questions about heart disease. The first part of Table 3.4 shows responses to the two questions that were asked of all respondents – whether they had ever had angina and whether they had ever had a heart attack 'including a heart murmur or a rapid heart'. The two questions overlap to some extent – someone with a heart attack may also have been diagnosed as having angina – and the questions showed a similar pattern of response when considered separately (see Nazroo, 1997a), consequently responses to them are combined in the table, which includes respondents who said that they had had either of these.

Overall as many as 4 per cent of ethnic minority people reported some form of diagnosed heart disease. However, the absolute per cents shown in Table 3.4 demonstrate that there was great variation between the different ethnic minority groups, with those in the Indian or African Asian group having the lowest rates, followed by the Caribbean group, and those in the Pakistani or Bangladeshi group having the highest rates. The difference between the two South Asian groupings has been partly documented elsewhere. Balarajan (1996) showed similar differences across the South Asian groups in his analysis of the most recent immigrant mortality data and there was a strong suggestion of a similar pattern in the 1999 Health Survey for England findings for diagnosed Ischaemic Heart Disease and ECG changes (Erens et al., 2001).

In comparison with the white group, the relative risk scores show a slightly lower rate for the Caribbean group and a substantially, and almost statistically significant, lower rate for the Indian or African Asian group. The relatively low rate for the Indian or African Asian group is surprising given the immigrant mortality data discussed in the introduction (Marmot et al., 1984; Balarajan, 1991 and 1996; Harding and Maxwell, 1997; Maxwell and Harding, 1998). Those in the Pakistani or Bangladeshi group, however, had much higher rates than the other groups, close to 50 per cent greater than that for the white group. This suggests the possibility that all of the difference reported elsewhere in coronary heart disease between South Asian and white people can be attributed to greater rates among the Pakistani and Bangladeshi groups.

The first section of Table 3.4 also shows that overall women reported lower rates of diagnosed heart disease than men, although this was not the case for those in the Caribbean group. There were no great differences in relative risk when comparing genders. Of all of the groups, Pakistani and Bangladeshi men reported particularly high rates of heart disease – around one in 15 Pakistani or Bangladeshi men reported that they had diagnosed heart disease. Given the age profiles of the Pakistani and Bangladeshi populations, this is not only a current serious health problem, but one that, as this population gets older, is likely to have very important consequences for these communities and health care provision (see also Lowy et al., 1991).

Of course, because they depend on respondents having consulted a doctor about cardiac symptoms and being aware of, understanding and remembering the diagnosis given, the questions on diagnosis may have undercounted prevalence and the undercounting may have varied across ethnic groups. In order to address this possibility, those who had not reported heart disease and who were aged 40 or more were asked additional questions on the experience of chest pain. An introductory question simply asked whether the respondent had experienced any chest pain. This was followed by a question that asked about 'severe chest pain lasting more than half an hour', which is likely to be more useful in terms of reflecting actual ischaemic heart disease. The second half of Table 3.4 combines the question asking about severe chest pain with those asking about diagnosed heart disease.

This follows a similar pattern to the results shown in the first half of the table for diagnosed heart disease only. The absolute per cent columns show that those in the Pakistani or Bangladeshi group had the highest rates among the ethnic minority groups, followed by the Caribbean group, with the Indian or African Asian group having the lowest rate (which was around half that of the Pakistani or Bangladeshi group). The age-standardised relative risks, calculated in comparison with the white group, for diagnosed heart disease or severe chest pain also show a similar pattern to those for diagnosed heart disease alone. Those in the Caribbean and Indian or African Asian groups had a rate very similar to that for the white group, while those in the Pakistani or Bangladeshi group had a rate that was much higher: over 80 per cent greater

## Table 3.4    Heart disease

| | White | Indian or African Asian | | Pakistani or Bangladeshi | | Caribbean | |
|---|---|---|---|---|---|---|---|
| | Absolute % | Absolute % | Age-standardised relative risk | Absolute % | Age-standardised relative risk | Absolute % | Age-standardised relative risk |
| **Diagnosed angina or heart attack[1]** | | | | | | | |
| Men | 8.0 | 4.1 | 0.83 (0.56-1.22) | 6.4 | 1.42 (1.02-1.99) | 4.3 | 0.67 (0.40-1.12) |
| Women | 6.2 | 2.5 | 0.72 (0.45-1.15) | 3.8 | 1.41 (0.94-2.09) | 4.3 | 1.21 (0.77-1.90) |
| Total | 7.0 | 3.3 | 0.79 (0.59-1.06) | 5.1 | 1.43 (1.11-1.84) | 4.3 | 0.88 (0.63-1.23) |
| *Unweighted base* | *2864* | *1998* | | *1773* | | *1202* | |
| **Diagnosed heart disease or severe chest pain[2]** | | | | | | | |
| Men | 19.0 | 12.5 | 0.83 (0.62-1.12) | 24.5 | 1.55 (1.21-2.00) | 15.8 | 0.78 (0.53-1.13) |
| Women | 14.2 | 11.9 | 1.10 (0.79-1.53) | 22.7 | 2.31 (1.74-3.08) | 14.2 | 1.27 (0.89-1.81) |
| Total | 16.3 | 12.2 | 0.93 (0.75-1.16) | 23.7 | 1.83 (1.52-2.21) | 14.9 | 0.96 (0.74-1.24) |
| *Unweighted base* | *1592* | *822* | | *590* | | *494* | |

1 In addition to 'heart attack', the question wording added 'including a heart murmur, a damaged heart or a rapid heart'.
2 Only those aged 40 or older are included here.

than that for any of the other ethnic groups. Interestingly, the rate for a combined South Asian grouping was 25 per cent higher than that for the white group, consistent with mortality data (Nazroo, 1997a, 2001).

These data confirm previous findings that suggest that South Asian people as a whole have higher rates of coronary heart disease than white people (Marmot et al., 1984; Balarajan, 1991 and 1996; Harding and Maxwell, 1997; Maxwell and Harding, 1998; Erens et al., 2001), but they also suggest that all of this difference can be attributed to higher rates among those in the Pakistani or Bangladeshi group. In fact, the white and Indian or African Asian groups seemed to have almost identical rates of coronary heart disease. The result seems robust in that it is repeated at each stage in the questioning, from questions addressing experience of symptoms to those asking about diagnosed heart disease, and across age (discussed next) and gender groups.

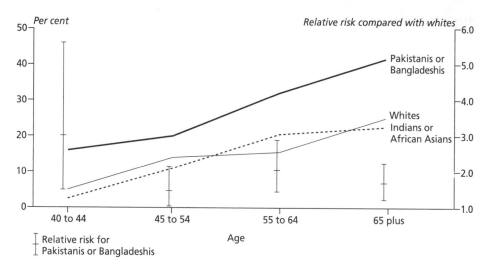

Figure 3.2   **Diagnosed heart disease or severe chest pain by age: white and South Asian groups**

Others have reported that the differences between South Asian and white people in mortality from heart disease are particularly large for the young (Balarajan, 1991). This is explored in Figure 3.2, which shows absolute per cents reporting diagnosed heart disease or severe chest pain for the two South Asian and the white group for four age categories. It also shows relative risks with 95 per cent confidence limits for the Pakistani or Bangladeshi group compared with the white group. The overall pattern remains similar to that shown in Table 3.4. Those in the Indian or African Asian group had the same rate as white people across the age categories and those in the Pakistani or Bangladeshi group had a higher rate than white people. The relative risk for Pakistani or Bangladeshi people was particularly large for those aged 40–44, being three times the white rate. However, absolute risk was greatest for the oldest age category, those aged 65 or more, where the difference between the Pakistani or Bangladeshi and white groups was more than 15 per cent.

In terms of the prevalence of possible coronary heart disease among ethnic minority groups, the results are a cause of great concern. Among those aged 40 or more, almost one in six people in ethnic minority groups reported heart disease or severe chest pain, while among the Pakistani or Bangladeshi group this figure was one in four. Even if we ignore the reports of severe chest pain, one in ten people in ethnic minority groups aged 40 or more reported that they had diagnosed heart disease, and this rose to one in seven among the Pakistani or Bangladeshi group. This clearly has very serious implications for both the ethnic minority communities concerned and the health service.

# Hypertension

Respondents were asked if they had ever suffered from hypertension and overall 11 per cent of people in ethnic minority groups reported they had. The absolute per cent columns in Table 3.5 show that the responses to this question varied across the ethnic minority groups in the way that would be predicted on the basis of published findings from immigrant mortality data (Marmot et al., 1984; Balarajan, 1991; Harding and Maxwell, 1997), with those in the Caribbean group having the highest rates. Overall one in five of the Caribbean group reported that they had hypertension, but the figures show an important gender difference. Close to one in four of the Caribbean women reported hypertension compared with just under one in six men.

The relative risk scores shown in the table also broadly confirm other studies on ethnic differences in hypertension. Compared with the white group, the Indian or African Asian group had significantly lower rates, the Pakistani or Bangladeshi group had similar rates, and the Caribbean group had rates almost 50 per cent higher. However, the relatively high rate for Caribbean respondents showed an interesting gender variation. For men, the Caribbean rate was only slightly and not significantly higher than the white rate, while for women the Caribbean rate was almost 80 per cent higher than the white rate. Similar findings are present in the 1999 Health Survey for England, which used measured rather than self-reported hypertension (Erens et al., 2001). Immigrant mortality data also suggest that the difference between women born in the Caribbean and women born in the UK is greater than that between men born in the Caribbean and men born in the UK (Marmot et al., 1984; Balarajan and Bulusu, 1990), but, unlike the data presented here and in the 1999 Health Survey for England, the mortality data do still reveal a difference between men.

## Table 3.5    Hypertension

| | White | Indian or African Asian | | Pakistani or Bangladeshi | | Caribbean | |
|---|---|---|---|---|---|---|---|
| | Absolute % | Absolute % | Age-standardised relative risk | Absolute % | Age-standardised relative risk | Absolute % | Age-standardised relative risk |
| **Diagnosed hypertension** | | | | | | | |
| Men | 15.0 | 10.2 | 0.88 (0.69-1.13) | 7.2 | 0.75 (0.58-0.98) | 14.6 | 1.12 (0.85-1.48) |
| Women | 16.7 | 5.8 | 0.46 (0.35-0.62) | 11.6 | 1.07 (0.87-1.34) | 22.7 | 1.79 (1.47-2.18) |
| Total | 15.9 | 8.0 | 0.66 (0.55-0.79) | 9.3 | 0.91 (0.77-1.08) | 19.1 | 1.47 (1.25-1.72) |
| *Unweighted base* | *2862* | *1994* | | *1770* | | *1195* | |

The data presented on hypertension clearly need to be treated with some caution. Hypertension is an asymptomatic condition and we have no knowledge of undiagnosed hypertension in this sample, nor how the process of diagnosis may be associated with both gender and ethnicity. It certainly seems possible that the routine checks for hypertension carried out on women in family planning and antenatal clinics will increase detection rates of hypertension for them compared with men, and this may partly explain the differences in both absolute per cents and relative risks shown for men and women in the Caribbean group. However, it is also worth noting that this gender difference is not reported consistently across the other ethnic groups in the table and that the findings do match those for measured hypertension in the 1999 Health Survey for England (Erens et al., 2001).

## DIABETES

All respondents were asked whether they had ever had diabetes. The relative risk scores in Table 3.6 show that all of the ethnic minority groups had higher rates of diabetes than the white group, although the size of the difference varied across the groups. Members of the Indian or African Asian and Caribbean groups had similarly high rates, about three times the white rate. Those in the Pakistani or Bangladeshi group had much higher rates than those in any other group, over five times the white rate.

Additional questions on type of diabetes were not asked, so distinctions could not be made between insulin dependent and non-insulin dependent diabetes (although the former is relatively rare), nor can those who only had diabetes during pregnancy be identified. In terms of the hypothesis relating insulin resistance to coronary heart disease (McKeigue et al., 1989), it is, of

Table 3.6    Diabetes

| | White | Indian or African Asian | | Pakistani or Bangladeshi | | Caribbean | |
|---|---|---|---|---|---|---|---|
| | Absolute % | Absolute % | Age-standardised relative risk | Absolute % | Age-standardised relative risk | Absolute % | Age-standardised relative risk |
| **Diagnosed diabetes** | | | | | | | |
| Men | 3.2 | 5.7 | 2.36 (1.52-3.68) | 7.8 | 3.84 (2.53-5.81) | 5.0 | 1.79 (1.04-3.08) |
| Women | 1.5 | 4.1 | 3.59 (2.05-6.27) | 6.9 | 7.76 (4.63-13.0) | 6.1 | 5.27 (3.02-9.22) |
| Total | 2.3 | 4.9 | 2.77 (1.97-3.89) | 7.4 | 5.24 (3.82-7.18) | 5.6 | 3.12 (2.16-4.50) |
| *Unweighted base* | *2862* | *2000* | | *1772* | | *1199* | |

course, impossible to identify with survey research of this kind whether reported diabetes is a result of insulin resistance or not. Like other reports of specific illness, it is again worth pointing out that responses to the diabetes question were dependent on the respondent consulting a doctor about possible symptoms and being aware of the diagnosis made.

## RESPIRATORY DISEASE

Half of the ethnic minority and all of the white respondents were asked several questions from the Medical Research Council respiratory questionnaire (MRC, 1982) in an attempt to identify possible respiratory illness. All of this questioning was around symptoms rather than diagnosis (which would have been very difficult to collect given both the number of sub-categories of diagnosis that could be given and the complexity of accurate diagnostic procedures) and many of the questions used could have been answered positively by those with breathlessness as a result of heart failure. Consequently, the data presented in Table 3.7 are based on an index of positive responses to the questions that should be most likely to be related to respiratory disease – wheezing or coughing up phlegm on most days for at least three months a year (respiratory symptoms).

Overall 18 per cent of both men and women in ethnic minority groups reported respiratory symptoms, with particularly high rates (close to one in four) among the Caribbean group. Not shown in the table is that there were only small gender differences in reporting these symptoms, although in the Pakistani or Bangladeshi group women had lower rates than men and in the Caribbean group men had lower rates than women. In comparison with the white group, the relative risks shown in the total row of Table 3.7 show that those in both of the South Asian groupings had a markedly lower risk of reporting respiratory symptoms than white people. (Interestingly, most of this difference related to the question on wheezing rather than that on coughing up phlegm.) Those in the Caribbean group, however, had a similar risk to white people.

There are important differences in rates of smoking across ethnic group, which have been documented elsewhere (Rudat, 1994) and are described in full for the Fourth National Survey in the next section of this chapter. It is possible that the low risk of respiratory symptoms among those in the South Asian groups shown in the total row of Table 3.7 is the result of their relatively low rates of smoking. This is explored in the smokers and non-smokers rows of the table. A comparison of the absolute per cents in these rows shows that smokers were much more likely than non-smokers to report respiratory symptoms in all groups. And the relative risk scores show that smokers in the South Asian groups were just as likely as white smokers to have reported respiratory symptoms; the lower risk for the South Asian groups only applied to non-smokers.

**Table 3.7    Respiratory symptoms**

| | White | Indian or African Asian | | Pakistani or Bangladeshi | | Caribbean | |
|---|---|---|---|---|---|---|---|
| | Absolute % | Absolute % | Age-standardised relative risk | Absolute % | Age-standardised relative risk | Absolute % | Age-standardised relative risk |
| **Wheezing or coughing up phlegm** | | | | | | | |
| Total | 28.1 | 14.5 | 0.55 (0.47-0.64) | 16.7 | 0.67 (0.57-0.78) | 23.5 | 0.87 (0.75-1.02) |
| Non-smokers | 22.0 | 12.3 | 0.59 (0.48-0.74) | 14.7 | 0.76 (0.61-0.94) | 21.1 | 1.05 (0.83-1.33) |
| Smokers | 33.9 | 31.1 | 1.03 (0.80-1.31) | 25.4 | 0.88 (0.70-1.11) | 27.9 | 0.85 (0.69-1.05) |
| *Unweighted base* | *2867* | *988* | | *873* | | *614* | |

## SMOKING

Half of the ethnic minority and all of the white respondents were asked questions on smoking, which covered both past and current smoking habits. Those respondents who said that they smoked one or more cigarettes per day were classified as regular smokers. Findings for ever having regularly smoked or currently regularly smoking are shown in Table 3.8. The patterns for ever and current smoking were very similar: among the ethnic minority groups those in the Caribbean group had the highest overall rates, followed by those in the Pakistani or Bangladeshi group, with the Indian or African Asian group having the lowest rates. These rates are similar to, although slightly higher than, the findings reported by Rudat (1994) and similar to, though slightly lower than, the findings reported for the 1999 Health Survey for England (Erens et al., 2001).

In comparison with the white group, the relative risk scores for all of the ethnic minority groups showed that they were significantly less likely to have ever been regular smokers, although differences were much more marked for the two South Asian groupings. This difference in comparison with the white group was still present, but smaller, for current regular smoking among the South Asian groupings. Those in the Caribbean group were just as likely as those in the white group to be current smokers.

The final row of the table shows the number of respondents who had been regular smokers, but were not currently smoking. Of concern is that the relative risks in this row show that ethnic minority smokers are much, and significantly, less likely than their white counterparts to have successfully given up. Looking at the unstandardised absolute per cent columns shows

*Ethnicity, Class and Health*

**Table 3.8    Smoking**

| | White | Indian or African Asian | | Pakistani or Bangladeshi | | Caribbean | |
|---|---|---|---|---|---|---|---|
| | Absolute % | Absolute % | Age-standardised relative risk | Absolute % | Age-standardised relative risk | Absolute % | Age-standardised relative risk |
| **Ever smoked regularly[1]** | | | | | | | |
| Men | 59.8 | 20.5 | 0.37 (0.31-0.45) | 36.3 | 0.69 (0.60-0.78) | 42.6 | 0.78 (0.68-0.90) |
| Women | 45.1 | 3.9 | 0.09 (0.06-0.13) | 1.4 | 0.03 (0.02-0.07) | 30.7 | 0.70 (0.59-0.82) |
| Total | 51.7 | 11.8 | 0.23 (0.20-0.28) | 19.5 | 0.39 (0.34-0.45) | 36.1 | 0.74 (0.67-0.83) |
| **Currently smoke regularly[1]** | | | | | | | |
| Men | 26.9 | 16.3 | 0.58 (0.46-0.72) | 31.0 | 1.13 (0.96-1.33) | 33.6 | 1.21 (1.00-1.45) |
| Women | 25.6 | 2.9 | 0.10 (0.06-0.17) | 1.4 | 0.05 (0.02-0.11) | 25.7 | 0.90 (0.73-1.09) |
| Total | 26.2 | 9.3 | 0.32 (0.26-0.40) | 16.8 | 0.58 (0.49-0.68) | 29.3 | 1.05 (0.92-1.20) |
| Regular[1] smokers who have given up | 49.3 | 21.2 | 0.49 (0.35-0.71) | 13.8 | 0.35 (0.24-0.50) | 18.8 | 0.46 (0.35-0.60) |
| *Unweighted base* | *2867* | *988* | | *873* | | *614* | |

1 Regular is more than one a day.

that while one in two white smokers had given up, only around one in five smokers in the Indian or African Asian and Caribbean groups had given up, and less than one in seven smokers in the Pakistani or Bangladeshi group had given up.

For all of the ethnic groups covered in the table, men were more likely than women to have reported ever smoking, but this was particularly marked for the South Asian groups, among whom very few women reported that they smoked. For current smoking, differences between men and women were maintained for all of the ethnic minority groups, if somewhat reduced for the Caribbean group, but had disappeared for the white group. The combination of those with Pakistani and Bangladeshi family origins into one group in this table obscures the particularly high rates of smoking among Bangladeshi men – 44 per cent of Bangladeshi men reported being current regular smokers and less than one in ten Bangladeshi men who had ever been regular smokers had given up.

# NEUROTIC DEPRESSION

Table 3.9 shows the estimated weekly prevalence for neurotic depression, an estimate that was based on the correlation between the CIS-R score and the chance of meeting the CATEGO criteria for the neurotic depression class, as shown in Chapter 2. The absolute per cent columns show that on the whole the gender difference reported elsewhere in the literature (Bebbington, 1996; Nazroo et al., 1998) was present here, although for the Pakistani or Bangladeshi group it was reversed. Compared with the white group, the relative risk columns show that those in the Caribbean group had much and significantly higher rates. In contrast, the Indian or African Asian and the Bangladeshi or Pakistani groups had lower rates than the white group, although these differences were not statistically significant.

It is interesting to note that the differences between the two South Asian groups and the white group were more marked for women than for men. While women in the South Asian groups all had lower rates than white women, South Asian men had similar rates to those of the white men.

**Table 3.9    Depression**

| | White | Indian or African Asian | | Pakistani or Bangladeshi | | Caribbean | |
|---|---|---|---|---|---|---|---|
| | Absolute %[1] | Absolute %[1] | Age-standardised relative risk[2] | Absolute %[1] | Age-standardised relative risk[2] | Absolute %[1] | Age-standardised relative risk[2] |
| **Estimated weekly prevalence of depressive neurosis** | | | | | | | |
| Men | 3.1 | 2.4 | 0.85 | 3.2 | 1.14 | 5.4 | 1.90 |
| | (2.1-4.1) | (1.8-3.1) | (0.44-1.63) | (2.2-4.2) | (0.63-2.07) | (3.6-7.3) | (1.06-3.42) |
| Women | 4.7 | 3.2 | 0.64 | 2.8 | 0.55 | 6.3 | 1.28 |
| | (3.2-6.2) | (2.2-4.2) | ( 0.38-1.07) | (1.9-3.7) | (0.30-1.00) | (4.4-8.3) | (0.81-2.02) |
| Total | 4.0 | 2.8 | 0.71 | 3.0 | 0.76 | 5.9 | 1.50 |
| | (2.7-5.3) | (2.0-3.7) | (0.48-1.07) | (2.1-3.9) | (0.50-1.15) | (4.0-7.8) | (1.04-2.15) |
| *Unweighted base* | *2867* | *988* | | *873* | | *614* | |

1 In the per cent columns, figures in brackets represent 95 per cent confidence limits that account for sampling error at the follow-up stage of the study.
2 For relative risk, 95 per cent confidence intervals do not take into account sampling error at the follow-up stage of the study.

# NON-AFFECTIVE PSYCHOSIS

Table 3.10 shows findings for the estimated annual prevalence of non-affective psychotic disorders among the different ethnic groups. Again it is worth emphasising that this was not based on case identification, but on the

**Table 3.10   Non-affective psychosis**

| | White | Indian or African Asian | | Pakistani or Bangladeshi | | Caribbean | |
|---|---|---|---|---|---|---|---|
| | Absolute %[1] | Absolute %[1] | Age-standardised relative risk[2] | Absolute %[1] | Age-standardised relative risk[2] | Absolute %[1] | Age-standardised relative risk[2] |
| **Estimated annual prevalence of non-affective psychosis** | | | | | | | |
| Men | 0.8 | 0.6 | 0.71 | 0.5 | 0.55 | 1.0 | 1.12 |
| | (0.4-1.3) | (0.3-0.9) | (0.26-1.90) | (0.2-0.8) | (0.18-1.65) | (0.5-1.5) | (0.39-3.18) |
| Women | 0.7 | 0.6 | 0.80 | 0.6 | 0.76 | 1.7 | 2.23 |
| | (0.3-1.1) | (0.3- 0.9) | (0.31-2.08) | (0.3-0.8) | (0.27-2.14) | (0.8-2.7) | (1.01-4.93) |
| Total | 0.8 | 0.6 | 0.75 | 0.5 | 0.65 | 1.4 | 1.65 |
| | (0.4-1.2) | (0.3-0.9) | (0.38-1.49) | (0.2-0.8) | (0.30-1.37) | (0.6-2.1) | (0.88-3.01) |
| *Unweighted base* | *2867* | *2001* | | *1776* | | *1205* | |

1 In the per cent columns, figures in brackets represent 95 per cent confidence limits that account for sampling error at the follow-up stage of the study.
2 For relative risk, 95 per cent confidence intervals do not take into account sampling error at the follow-up stage of the study.

correlation between the PSQ score and the chance of meeting the CATEGO criteria for a psychotic class, as shown in Chapter 2. The rate for the white group should be comparable to the general population rate reported in the National Psychiatric Morbidity Survey (Meltzer et al., 1995), but is twice that. If the conservative method of case finding used in the National Psychiatric Morbidity Survey is used here (see Chapter 2), the estimate rates become comparable, with a rate of 0.36 per cent in the Fourth National Survey white group compared with the National Psychiatric Morbidity Survey general population estimate of 0.4 per cent with a standard error of 0.1 per cent.[1]

The relative risk columns show that overall those in the Caribbean group had a rate that was two-thirds higher than that of the white group. In contrast, overall those in the Indian or African Asian and Pakistani or Bangladeshi groups had rates that were lower than for the white group. None of these differences was statistically significant. Although the sample size was sufficiently large for statistical tests to detect the three to five times greater rate of psychosis among the Caribbean compared with the white group that would be expected on the basis of previous research, it was not sufficiently large for statistical tests to identify differences of the size reported here, so the lack of statistical significance should be interpreted with caution.

---

1    Differences between the two surveys may also have been a result of the different instruments used. Here the PSE 9 (based on ICD8) was used to identify cases, while in the National Psychiatric Morbidity Survey the PSE 10 (based on ICD10) was used.

The table shows interesting gender effects for the Caribbean group. Women in the Caribbean group had more than twice the estimated rate of white women (a difference that was statistically significant), while Caribbean men had a rate that was close to that for white British men. Also, not shown in the table is that the data showed no clear age effects. There was a tendency for the prevalence to decrease with age for the white group, but not for the Caribbean group, and it possibly increased with age for those in the Indian or African Asian and Pakistani or Bangladeshi groups. Even if smaller age categories are considered for the Caribbean group, there was no evidence that a cohort effect, as would be predicted by Glover's (1989) hypothesis, was present in this sample.

## CONCLUSION

The Fourth National Survey was the first fully representative assessment of the health of ethnic minority groups in England and Wales. Consequently, the data presented in this chapter provide a benchmark against which health needs can be assessed, changes determined, and comparisons between ethnic groups made.

The data illustrate important differences between ethnic minority and white groups in reported health. They broadly confirm differences suggested by other studies based on morbidity and mortality data. However, there are also some important discrepancies between the data presented here and conclusions reached elsewhere. As far as general health is concerned, the data indicate that those in the Pakistani or Bangladeshi groups were particularly disadvantaged compared with white people, having a 50 per cent greater risk of reported fair, poor, or very poor health (see Table 3.1), and over twice the risk of having their performance of moderately exerting activities limited by their health (see Table 3.3). Members of the Caribbean group were also disadvantaged compared with the white group, being about 30 per cent more likely to have reported fair, poor, or very poor health or that their performance of moderately exerting activities was limited by their health. Although previous research has indicated that all ethnic minority groups have poorer general health than white people (Benzeval et al., 1992; Pilgrim et al., 1993; Williams et al., 1993; Rudat, 1994), here differences between those in the Indian or African Asian and white groups were small and not statistically significant. This discrepancy may be a result of more effective sampling in this survey – the sample used here is nationally representative rather than either reflecting a local situation or only being drawn from areas with a relatively large ethnic minority population – and careful allocation of individuals into specific ethnic groups. The 1991 Census and the 1999 Health Survey for England also meet both of these criteria, and the questions on limiting long-standing illness used in the Census and self-assessed general health and limiting long-standing illness in the 1999 Health Survey for

England (Erens et al., 2001) showed a very similar pattern of response to all but one of the indicators of general health used here (see Nazroo, 1997a, for full details of the Census findings).

The indicator of general health used here that did not follow the pattern of the others, or that of the census, was whether the respondent reported any long-standing illness. The Indian or African Asian and Pakistani or Bangladeshi groups did significantly better on this indicator than the white group, and those in the Caribbean group had the same rate as white people (see Table 3.2). Evidence presented here and elsewhere (Pilgrim et al., 1993) suggests that this may be due to problems with the use of such a question for making comparisons across ethnic groups, unless its phrasing includes some notion of the illness limiting the respondent in some way – see the contradictory pattern for long-standing illness limiting work (also found in Table 3.2).

Interestingly, the ethnic differences in response to general health questions did not begin to emerge until above the age of 35; for those aged 16 to 34 there were no, or minimal, differences between ethnic groups. This may be a result of the very low rates of ill-health in this age group (Blane et al., 1994), or because ethnic differences in the key forms of material, cultural or biological disadvantage that are related to poor health do not emerge until early middle age.

Immigrant mortality data suggest that those born in South Asia have higher rates of coronary heart disease than those born in Britain and that those born in the Caribbean have lower rates (Marmot et al., 1984; Balarajan 1991 and 1996; Harding and Maxwell, 1997; Maxwell and Harding, 1998). The morbidity data presented here also indicate that those in the Caribbean group had lower rates of coronary heart disease than white people, although differences were not statistically significant. Of the South Asian groups, somewhat unexpectedly those in the Indian or African Asian group appeared to have similar rates of coronary heart disease to those in the white group. However, members of the Pakistani or Bangladeshi group had considerably higher rates of coronary heart disease than those in the white group according to the measures used in this survey. Examining differences between the Pakistani or Bangladeshi and white groups by age showed a pattern that was consistent with the differences in age-related mortality that are reported between those born in the Indian sub-continent and those born in Britain.

When considering the differences between the morbidity data presented here and the mortality data presented elsewhere, it is important to keep in mind three factors. First, as described in Chapter 1, ethnicity for mortality data is not adequately collected, being based on country of birth, so real differences in mortality rates between the various South Asian groups may not have been identified by previous studies. Indeed, the data presented by Balarajan et al. (1984) suggest that Muslims may have higher mortality rates from ischaemic heart disease than others born in the Indian sub-continent, and the more recent immigrant mortality data presented by Balarajan (1996) and morbidity data from the 1999 Health Survey for England (Erens et al.,

2001) suggest that those born in Bangladesh and Pakistan have higher rates of mortality and morbidity from heart disease than those born in India.

Second, this discrepancy might be related to measurement problems; for example, heart disease may be over-recorded as a cause of death for those born in South Asia, or Indian or African Asian people may have under-reported heart disease morbidity in this survey. There are clearly potential problems with both the sensitivity and specificity of the questions used, which may vary across ethnic groups. Unfortunately, no evidence on this is available in the data reported. However, the findings do show a remarkable consistency in response across the different types of questions used to identify heart disease, as well as the expected variation in rate across gender and age for each group. Elsewhere, there is only limited evidence on differences in response to questions on heart disease across social groups. One study, using a vignette, has suggested that South Asian and white people interpret chest pain similarly (Chaturvedi et al., 1997). Others have suggested that socio-economic position might be related to the under-reporting of symptoms more generally (Blane et al., 1996; Mackenback et al., 1996).

Third, mortality rates and reported morbidity rates do not necessarily co-vary. As a result of differences in access to treatment, or in the natural progression of the disease, or in exposure to environmental or social factors which may influence the progression of the disease, coronary heart morbidity may well lead to different rates of mortality among different social groups. Indeed, rates of survival following myocardial infarction have been shown to vary for both socio-economic group (Morrison et al., 1997) and for ethnic group, with South Asian people appearing to have lower survival rates than white comparisons (Wilkinson et al., 1996; Shaukat et al., 1997).[2] This may be partly a consequence of differences in treatment. It has been shown that among those suffering a myocardial infarction, rates of admission to hospital are related to area deprivation scores (Morrison et al., 1997), that South Asians with CHD wait longer for referral to specialist care than whites (Shaukat et al., 1993) and, among those who have suffered an acute myocardial infarction, one study has suggested that Indian patients are less likely to be treated with thrombolysis, or to be referred for exercise stress tests (Lear et al., 1994a and 1994b). Another suggested that they are less likely to receive coronary bypass surgery (Shaukat et al., 1997). In addition, ethnic differences in the progression of the disease might be important. In another study, although white and South Asian patients admitted to hospital with a myocardial infarction received very similar treatment, the South Asian patients had a higher case fatality rate than the white patients, perhaps because of a higher co-morbidity with diabetes (Wilkinson et al., 1996).

---

2  Interestingly, the two papers showing higher mortality rates for South Asian compared with white people following a myocardial infarct favoured different explanations. Shaukat et al. (1997) based their explanation on the presence of more extensive arterial disease, while Wilkinson et al. (1996) suggested that differences were a consequence of greater co-morbidity with diabetes.

Fourth, there may be important cohort differences between the populations included in the immigrant mortality data collected over the past two decades and those included in this morbidity survey carried out in 1993 and 1994. Indeed, there is some suggestion of a possible cohort effect in a recently published comparison of immigrant mortality statistics from 1970–72 with those from 1989–92, with men born in South Asia having a Standardised Mortality Rate of 183 (95 per cent confidence intervals 172 to 193) for the earlier period and 146 (95 per cent confidence intervals 141 to 162) for the later period (Wild and McKeigue, 1997).

The data presented on rates of hypertension confirm previous findings of higher rates of mortality related to hypertension among those born in the Caribbean compared with those born in Britain (Marmot et al., 1984; Balarajan and Bulusu, 1990). Among the South Asian respondents in this sample, the rate of hypertension for those in the Indian or African Asian group was lower than that for the white group, while it was about the same as the white group for those in the Pakistani or Bangladeshi group. Although this is consistent with the measured hypertension data from the 1999 Health Survey for England (Erens et al., 2001), this is again in contrast to data on immigrant mortality from hypertensive disease and mortality from strokes. These suggest that the South Asian groups should have higher rates of hypertension than the general population (Balarajan and Bulusu, 1990; Harding and Maxwell, 1997; Maxwell and Harding, 1998). Some of the explanations presented in the above paragraph may apply to this discrepancy. However, it is also worth noting that in a survey such as this the recognition of hypertension is totally dependent on diagnosis by a doctor. Different ethnic (and gender) groups may well have had different opportunities for such a diagnosis to be made.

In this sample, rates of diabetes showed the expected ethnic differences, with all of the ethnic minority groups having higher rates than the white group. Interestingly, the difference between the South Asian and white groups was much greater for Pakistani or Bangladeshi people than for Indian or African Asian people. Similar findings are present in the 1999 Health Survey for England (Erens et al., 2001).

Table 3.8 showed that white people are far more likely than the other groups to have reported ever regularly smoking, although differences for current smoking among men were smaller. One of the consequences of smoking is respiratory disease. For the indicators of respiratory disease used here (wheezing or coughing up phlegm), white people did worse than those in the other ethnic groups. This is consistent with immigrant mortality data (Marmot et al., 1984; Balarajan and Bulusu, 1990). However, if patterns of smoking are considered, among those who had ever regularly smoked, the size of ethnic differences in respiratory symptoms was much reduced and not significant, suggesting that the overall differences reported are largely a result of different patterns of smoking. This possibility is slightly weakened by the fact that there was a greater rate of respiratory symptoms among white non-smokers compared with non-smokers in the South Asian groups, although this may be the result of differences in exposure to passive smoking.

Ethnic inequalities in neurotic and psychotic disorders were estimated using responses to the CIS-R and PSQ questionnaires, some of which were validated in a follow-up clinical interview using the PSE (the full details of this are described in Chapter 2). Overall, a very similar pattern of findings was present for both neurotic depression and non-affective psychosis. Compared with the white group, for both of these outcomes those in the Caribbean group had higher rates, while members of the Indian or African Asian and Pakistani or Bangladeshi groups had lower rates.

However, this pattern was not entirely consistent for men and women. For the South Asian groups, rates of neurotic disorder were particularly low for women. Indeed, for men in the Pakistani or Bangladeshi group they were, if anything, higher than those for the white group. For the Caribbean group a similar pattern to that for the South Asian groups was present for neurotic disorders, with the rates for men being much greater and the rates for women being only slightly greater than those for equivalent white respondents. For psychosis there was also a significant gender variation in relative rates for the Caribbean group, with rates for females being over twice those of women in the white group and rates for Caribbean males being almost the same as those for men in the white group. The higher rate of psychosis that was present for the Caribbean group was not as large as might have been expected on the basis of previous work in this area (Bagley, 1971; McGovern and Cope, 1987; Harrison et al., 1988; Littlewood and Lipsedge, 1988; Cochrane and Bal, 1989; van Os et al., 1996). It was also entirely restricted to women and showed no evidence of a cohort or age effect. In addition, rates of depression were higher for the Caribbean compared with the white group, while previous work has suggested that they should be lower (Cochrane and Bal, 1989).

Some caveats need to be added to the interpretation of the findings on mental health. First, as shown in Chapter 2, the validation process did not perform uniformly across all groups. Indeed, there was a strong suggestion that the measures of depressive disorder did not perform adequately for the South Asian groups and, as described earlier, this may have led to an underestimation of rates for these groups. Alternatively, the strategy of ignoring ethnic differences in confirmation rates during the follow-up phase of the study, which was adopted here when estimating rates of depression, may have led to an overestimation of rates of depression for the South Asian groups and minimised genuine differences between ethnic groups. The possibilities of under- and overestimation will be explored more fully when language and migration effects are considered in Chapter 5, but the figures on depression for respondents in the South Asian groups reported in this chapter should be regarded with caution.

Second, as for depression, the estimated prevalence of psychosis depends on the assumption that the PSQ instrument performed reasonably uniformly across ethnic groups, gender and age (and, for comparisons in later chapters, socio-economic position and marital status). However, as described earlier, as far as it was possible to determine this was the case, so variations in validation rates for the PSQ may not have been a serious problem.

Finally, it is worth restating one important issue that emerged from the data as far as gender is concerned. For many of the indicators of health, in the Caribbean group men did better than women when compared with their white counterparts. Differences for psychosis have just been described. The higher rate of ill-health among those in the Caribbean group compared with the white group according to most indicators of general health was the result of differences between Caribbean and white women. This also applied to differences in the rate of diagnosed hypertension, with Caribbean men having the same rate as white men and Caribbean women having much higher rates than white women.

# CHAPTER FOUR

# Exploring ethnic diversity further: differences in health across religious sub-groups

## INTRODUCTION

The use of overarching ethnic categories, such as 'all ethnic minorities' or 'South Asian', in research on ethnic differences in health has been widely criticised, because it combines distinct ethnic groups with different cultural traditions, migration experiences and socio-economic positions (Modood, 1994; Modood et al., 1997). The suggestion is that the use of overarching categories is misleading, because the constituents covered by such groupings have very diverse experiences. Indeed, tables presented in Chapter 3 showed that a simple division of those in the South Asian ethnic category into Indian or African Asian and Pakistani or Bangladeshi groups produced categories with very diverse health experiences. This, of course, is directly related to the wider criticisms of the basis of ethnic categorisations used in health research (Chaturvedi and McKeigue, 1994; McKenzie and Crowcroft, 1994 and 1996; Senior and Bhopal, 1994; Bradby, 1995), described in Chapter 2, and whether a meaningful categorisation of ethnic group should be theoretically or empirically driven. For example, similar criticisms could be levelled at the use throughout most of this volume of ethnic categories based on country of family origin. Although the division of the South Asian category into the two groups used in Chapter 3 made some *empirical* sense – Pakistani people had a very similar health profile to Bangladeshi people and Indian people had a very similar health profile to African Asian people (Nazroo, 1997a) – it is possible that an ethnic classification based on country of family origin is itself too crude to provide an adequate *theoretical* understanding. In particular, the Indian or African Asian category includes populations from distinct regions within India and Africa, and with different cultural traditions, migration histories and socio-economic positions. In fact, a unique study by Balarajan et al. (1984), which used an analysis of names to subdivide those born in India into regional and religious groups, demonstrates that such groups may well have different patterns of disease.

In this context, it is worth recognising that a number of local studies of South Asian people have, in fact, been studies of particular sub-groups within this Indian category (e.g. Williams et al.'s (1993) study of the Punjabi population in Glasgow, Cruikshank et al.'s (1991) study of glucose resistance in the predominantly Gujarati population of north-west London, and Mather and Keen's (1985) study of diabetes in the Punjabi population of Southall, London). Here, it is of concern that at least some of these regional studies have their findings generalised to a more global category, such as 'South Asian', with the implication that findings derived from quite specific populations are then interpreted as if they apply to all components of a much wider ethnic minority population.

So, the use of overarching ethnic categories allows researchers to ignore ethnic diversity, which potentially facilitates the reduction of ethnic groups to essential characteristics, and allows studies of particular constituencies within the overarching category to be generalised to all other constituencies within the category. In order to explore the implications of this further, in this chapter the ethnic category of Indian or African Asian will be subdivided to see whether important differences emerge between groups. The intention is to explore how useful it is to use geographical, cultural or religious markers to deconstruct ethnic categories that are based on country of family origin into ethnic 'sub-groupings'. In this survey this is most easily done with those respondents who described themselves as having Indian family origins, because they can be conveniently divided into three cultural/geographical groups: Hindus from the Gujarati region of India; Sikhs from the Punjabi region of India; and Muslims from a number of areas. Although this exercise will be carried out only on the Indian or African Asian group, the lessons that are learned can be generalised to other groups. In particular, if important differences do emerge between sub-groups in the Indian or African Asian category, this will also raise questions about the ethnic homogeneity of the other ethnic groupings that are used in health research, including the white, Caribbean, and Pakistani or Bangladeshi groups used here.

## Using the Fourth National Survey to compare the health of ethnic sub-groups in the Indian or African Asian category

For the purposes of the analysis carried out here, Indian and African Asian people will be considered jointly, as both groups describe their family origins as Indian and combining these groups gives a large enough sample size for such an analysis to be carried out. Also, as already described, these two groups have similar levels of ill-health across a variety of dimensions (Nazroo, 1997a). Religion will be used as the marker of ethnic sub-group within the Indian or African Asian category. This involves focusing on four main groups: Hindus; Sikhs; Muslims; and Christians. Other studies, which have used an analysis of names to determine ethnic (sub-) group, have tended to include Indian Christians in a white group on the basis that: 'Anglo-Indians and Indians with English names (mostly Christians) ... probably have a lifestyle similar to that of people of English descent' (Balarajan et al., 1984: 1185) and: 'Counting

**Table 4.1     Religion for Indian and African Asian people**

|  |  |  | *Column percentages* |
|---|---|---|---|
|  | Indian | African Asian | Total |
| **Religion** |  |  |  |
| Hindu | 33 | 58 | 42 |
| Sikh | 50 | 19 | 38 |
| Muslim | 6 | 15 | 9 |
| Christian | 5 | 3 | 4 |
| Other or none | 6 | 5 | 6 |
| *Unweighted base* | *(1273)* | *(728)* | *(2001)* |

'Anglo-Indian' as British is justified by their way of life and easy entry to the UK, governed as it is by having a British parent or grandparent' (Marmot et al., 1984: 9). This perspective clearly prejudges the explanatory focus of the analysis that is to be undertaken, i.e. that it will be based on lifestyle factors, and the field of interest of the research, i.e. it is about the 'Other'. When exploring the diversity of health experience among Indian people in Britain, it seems useful to include, rather than exclude, a group who describe their family origins as Indian and who are Christians.

It should be noted that the categories of Indian and African Asian are differentially related to religion. As shown in Table 4.1, Indian people were more likely to be Sikhs than African Asian people who, in turn, were more likely to be Hindus or Muslims. The table also shows that a small percentage of respondents in these ethnic groups said that they had no religion or a religion other than Hindu, Sikh, Muslim or Christian. This group will almost certainly be very heterogeneous in make-up, but is too small to be separated, and is, consequently, not considered in this chapter.

The comparisons between the religious groups presented in this section of the chapter have not been standardised for age and gender, because differences between the age and gender profiles of the group were only minor. However, it is worth bearing in mind that the Hindu group had slightly more men than the other groups (52 per cent compared with 50 per cent for all members of the Indian or African Asian group) and that the Sikh group was slightly younger than the other groups (median age for Sikhs was 34, compared with 36 for all those in the Indian or African Asian group).

## SELF-ASSESSED GENERAL HEALTH

Responses to the question asking the respondent to rate his or her health on a five-point scale ranging from very poor to excellent, which was asked of all respondents, are shown in Table 4.2. The table suggests that Muslims were

**Table 4.2    Reported health compared with others of the same age by religion for Indian and African Asian people**

|  |  |  |  | *Cell percentages* |
| --- | --- | --- | --- | --- |
|  | Hindu | Sikh | Muslim | Christian |
| Those reporting fair, poor, or very poor health | 26.9 | 28.2 | 31.6 | 26.0 |
| *Unweighted base* | *819* | *704* | *284* | *85* |

more likely to report that their health was fair, poor, or very poor than the other religious groups. However, the differences in the table are not statistically significant.

## HEART DISEASE

All respondents were asked whether they had had angina or 'a heart attack – including a heart murmur, a damaged heart or a rapid heart'. The first part of Table 4.3 includes respondents who said that they had had either of these. It shows that Muslims and Christians were more likely than others to have had diagnosed heart disease, and that Hindus were less likely.

In addition to questions on the diagnosis of heart disease, respondents aged 40 or more were asked questions about the experience of severe chest pain. The second part of Table 4.3 shows respondents who reported either diagnosed heart disease or severe chest pain. As for the diagnosed heart disease-only outcome,

**Table 4.3    Ischaemic heart disease by religion for Indian and African Asian people**

|  |  |  |  | *Cell percentages* |
| --- | --- | --- | --- | --- |
|  | Hindu | Sikh | Muslim | Christian |
| Diagnosed angina or heart attack[1] | 1.7[3] | 3.9 | 5.8[4] | 7.7[4] |
| *Unweighted base* | *819* | *706* | *285* | *85* |
| Diagnosed heart disease or severe chest pain[2] | 7.7[3] | 14.1 | 18.5[4] | 18.4 |
| *Unweighted base* | *345* | *285* | *111* | *41* |

1 In addition to 'heart attack', the question wording added 'including a heart murmur, a damaged heart or a rapid heart'.
2 Only those aged 40 or older are included here.
3 $p < 0.01$ compared with the other groups combined (1 d.f.).
4 $p < 0.05$ compared with the other groups combined (1 d.f.).

**Table 4.4 Hypertension by religion for Indian and African Asian people**

|  | Hindu[1] | Sikh | Muslim | Christian |
|---|---|---|---|---|
|  |  |  |  | *Cell percentages* |
| Diagnosed hypertension | 6.4 | 8.6 | 9.4 | 13.0 |
| *Unweighted base* | *819* | *702* | *284* | *85* |

1 p < 0.05 compared with the other groups combined (1 d.f.).

Muslims and Christians were more likely than others and Hindus were less likely than others to meet these criteria. Although the rate for the Christian and Muslim groups was similar, for the Christian group differences were not statistically significant (because of differences in sample size).

## OTHER SPECIFIC ILLNESSES

Table 4.4 shows the percentage of respondents who reported that they had hypertension. Although only the lower rate for Hindus was significant, there is also a suggestion that Christians were more likely than others to have had hypertension.

Table 4.5 shows that Christians were also more likely to have reported that they had diabetes and, unlike the situation for all of the other assessments of health reported in this section, Muslims were the least likely to have reported that they had diabetes. Again the differences shown in this table were not statistically significant.

**Table 4.5 Diabetes by religion for Indian and African Asian people**

|  | Hindu | Sikh | Muslim | Christian |
|---|---|---|---|---|
|  |  |  |  | *Cell percentages* |
| Diagnosed diabetes | 5.1 | 4.6 | 4.3 | 6.6 |
| *Unweighted base* | *819* | *707* | *285* | *85* |

Half of the respondents were asked whether they had had a variety of respiratory symptoms. Table 4.6 shows the percentage of respondents who were positive on an index of those questions that should be most likely to be related to respiratory disease – wheezing or coughing up phlegm on most days for at least three months a year (respiratory symptoms). Muslims were more likely and Christians were much less likely than others to have reported these symptoms, although again the differences were not statistically significant.

Table 4.6    **Respiratory symptoms by religion for Indian and African Asian people**

| | | | | *Cell percentages* |
|---|---|---|---|---|
| | Hindu | Sikh | Muslim | Christian |
| Wheezing or coughing up phlegm | 13.7 | 13.9 | 17.6 | 7.4 |
| *Unweighted base* | *407* | *344* | *139* | *39* |

## SMOKING

Half of the ethnic minority sample were asked questions on smoking. Table 4.7 shows the percentage of respondents who reported that they had ever smoked. Muslims were the most likely to report that they had smoked. Christians were also more likely than Hindus and Sikhs to have smoked. And Sikhs, whose religion is anti-smoking, were the least likely to say that they had smoked.

Table 4.7    **Smoking by religion for Indian and African Asian people**

| | | | | *Cell percentages* |
|---|---|---|---|---|
| | Hindu | Sikh | Muslim | Christian |
| Ever smoked | 13.2 | 5.8[1] | 20.1[1] | 47.9[1] |
| *Unweighted base* | *407* | *344* | *139* | *39* |

1 $p < 0.01$ compared with the other groups combined (1 d.f.).

## MENTAL ILLNESS

The first part of Table 4.8 shows differences in the estimated weekly prevalence of neurotic depression across the religious groups contained in the Indian or African Asian category. And the second part shows differences in the estimated annual prevalence of non-affective psychosis. (Both of these are estimated using the procedure and formulae shown in Chapter 2.)

Both sections of the table show a very similar pattern. Muslims and Christians had similarly high rates of both outcomes (Christians had slightly higher rates than Muslims in both cases), while Hindus and Sikhs had rates that were around half those of Christians and Muslims for both outcomes (Sikhs had rates slightly lower than those of Hindus in both cases). However, none of these differences is statistically significant.

**Table 4.8     Mental illness by religion for Indian and African Asian people**

| | | | | *Cell percentages* |
|---|---|---|---|---|
| | Hindu | Sikh | Muslim | Christian |
| Estimated weekly prevalence of depressive neurosis | 2.9 | 2.0 | 4.1 | 5.2 |
| *Unweighted base* | *406* | *344* | *137* | *39* |
| Estimated annual prevalence of non-affective psychosis | 0.6 | 0.4 | 1.1 | 1.3 |
| *Unweighted base* | *817* | *707* | *280* | *85* |

## CONCLUSION

This chapter has shown the extent of differences in health by religious group for those with Indian family origins (those who elsewhere in this volume are described as Indian or African Asian). The most striking differences were found for heart disease. Both Muslims and Christians reported higher rates of diagnosed heart disease than Hindus and Sikhs, and this finding was repeated when, for those age 40 or older, either diagnosed heart disease or severe chest pain was considered. Other assessments of health did not show statistically significant differences between groups. However, all but one, whether the respondent reported having diabetes, suggested that Muslims had worse health than Hindus and Sikhs. And most suggested that Christians also had poorer health than Hindus or Sikhs. The consistency of this result across a variety of health indicators, together with the relatively small sample size of Muslims (285 respondents when the full sample is considered and 139 when half the sample is considered) and Christians (85 respondents when the full sample is considered and 39 when half the sample is considered), suggests that there are genuine differences in the health of these groups. Indeed, an inflexible interpretation of the lack of statistical significance for these health indicators (except those assessing heart disease) could lead to type II errors being made (where genuine differences are ignored (Blalock, 1985)).

The only item of health-related behaviour shown here, smoking, also had striking differences between the religious groups. Christians were the most likely ever to have smoked – one in two said that they had smoked – followed by Muslims – one in five Muslims said that they had smoked. Rates of smoking among Hindus and Sikhs were both low – about one in eight Hindus and only one in seventeen Sikhs said that they had smoked.

Returning to the issues that were raised in the introduction to this chapter, what is clear from these data is that considering ethnic groupings as internally homogeneous – whether the categorisation used is based on continent of birth, country of birth, country of family origin, or self-identification – is potentially misleading. Evidence presented here confirms the conclusion that important differences in both health and health behaviour can be found within these broad ethnic groupings when smaller ethnic groups are considered. This is potentially of great significance for epidemiological approaches to aetiological understanding, relying as they do on the ability to make comparisons across social groupings to identify those at higher risk of an adverse outcome (Marmot et al., 1984; Senior and Bhopal, 1994). It does, however, remain unclear whether the use of finer indicators of ethnic boundaries in such work is of great theoretical, or policy, value, when explanatory factors are unmeasured and assumptions are made about the genetic or cultural basis of differences across ethnic groups (Sheldon and Parker, 1992; Ahmad, 1996). It is not clear whether more refined measures of ethnicity will improve our understanding, or increase the ease with which explanations for ethnic differences in health are reduced to stereotyped characteristics of essentialised ethnic groups. This debate will be returned to in the conclusion.

# CHAPTER FIVE

# Migration and ethnic differences in health

## INTRODUCTION

On the whole, in this book responses to a question on country of family origin have been used to explore ethnic differences in health. This has considerable advantages over the use of country of birth as a proxy for ethnicity, which most other national studies have been forced to rely on (e.g. Marmot et al., 1984; Balarajan, 1991 and 1996; Harding and Maxwell, 1997; Wild and McKeigue, 1997; Maxwell and Harding, 1998), but, as illustrated in Chapter 4, it is itself not without disadvantages. Although these issues and their implications have been discussed in part in previous chapters and will be returned to in the conclusion to this volume, in the light of the contrasts between the findings presented in Chapter 3 and immigrant mortality rates, it is worth further exploring issues relating to migration *per se*.

In fact, a significant number of ethnic minority respondents to the Fourth National Survey were born in Britain, which gives the opportunity to provide a comparison between those born in Britain and those who had migrated to Britain. In addition to allowing an exploration of the implications of using country of birth as a surrogate ethnic classification, and how far this may have resulted in the discrepancies between the findings reported here and published data on immigrant mortality rates, such a comparison will also allow an exploration of how far issues related to migration might contribute to ethnic inequalities in health.

## The relationship between migration and health

There have been a number of discussions of how the process of migration could be directly related to health. These clearly have implications both for the interpretation of data that use country of birth to allocate ethnic group and, given the large number of migrants among the ethnic minority populations of Britain, for the interpretation of ethnic differences in health in studies that have used more appropriate assessments of ethnicity.

The first issue of relevance here is a consideration of how health may be related to the selection of individuals into a migrant group. Migrants may well differ from non-migrants in their country of origin in a number of ways, including age, gender and socio-economic position. Many of these factors will be related to health and if, as seems possible, migrants are younger and better educated than those who remain, they will have better health. The Nuffield Social Mobility Survey found that nearly a quarter of non-white migrants to Britain had professional class origins (Heath and Ridge, 1983).

In addition, health itself may be one of the factors that differs between the migrant and non-migrant populations of a country. On the one hand, those who are in poor health may, because of the difficulties they will face, be less likely to migrate than those who are healthy – a 'healthy migrant' effect. In support of this possibility, Marmot et al. (1984) presented data that suggested that migrants to England and Wales from all countries where comparisons could be made (which, unfortunately, did not include the Indian sub-continent), with the exception of Ireland, had a lower mortality rate than those in their country of birth – although there are a number of competing explanations for this finding. Alternatively, migration may be inversely related to health. Marmot et al. (1984) suggested that migrants to England and Wales from Ireland did not follow the pattern described above for two reasons. First, geographical and political differences in the process of migration for Irish people meant that they did not face a health barrier when migrating, so, rather than migrants being selected from the more advantaged groups in Ireland, they may have been selected from the more disadvantaged groups[1] who, of course, had poorer health. Indeed, it seems quite possible that those who are more marginal in society and, consequently, more disadvantaged will be more likely to migrate if an opportunity arises. Second, poor health itself may directly lead to migration – perhaps as a result of exclusion from the society of birth, because of the presence of a stigmatising illness, or possibly in search of better health care. There is, however, little empirical evidence beyond Heath and Ridge's (1983) work to support any of these possibilities. It is also the case that where whole communities have been forced to migrate, as happened to South Asian people living in East Africa in the late 1960s and early 1970s, neither negative nor positive health selection would have played a role in the process of migration (although it may have influenced the migrant's choice of country).

The second issue that needs consideration is the direct effect of the process of migration on health. Migration involves a great deal of social disruption and stress. Social networks break down and are often re-formed in new and unexpected ways (Khan, 1979). This will have implications for the extent and nature of the social support that exists in migrant communities. There will also be changes in economic position and economic opportunity once migration has occurred, and the movement into an unfamiliar and probably hostile environment will undoubtedly cause considerable stress. All of these factors

---

1    Differences in the socio-economic pressures to migrate in the country of origin presumably also played a role in determining different patterns of migration to Britain.

may have an adverse impact on the health of migrant ethnic minority populations.

The third issue that is of relevance here is the importance of environmental experiences on health. The impact of environmental factors during childhood on adult health is a topic that has raised considerable interest (Barker, 1991; Vågerö and Illsley, 1995) and this may be of particular relevance to ethnic inequalities in health. It certainly seems possible that greater environmental deprivation in the country of birth for migrants compared with others is one of the explanatory factors for the ethnic inequalities in health that have been demonstrated in immigrant mortality studies. In support of this, Williams et al. (1993) concluded that differences in the physical development of members of the Punjabi population in Glasgow compared with the white population were the result of childhood environmental deprivation in the Punjab. If this is the case, we would expect ethnic inequalities in health to diminish as new generations are born in Britain. In fact, there is some evidence from the US to suggest that within one or two generations the health of ethnic minority populations becomes similar to that of others in the country to which they migrated (e.g. Syme et al., 1975; Gordon, 1982). This supports the possibility that ethnic inequalities in health are a consequence of differences in environmental risk in different countries of birth. In contrast, at least part of the explanation for the reported high rates of psychosis among *British-born* African Caribbean people (McGovern and Cope, 1987; Harrison et al., 1988) compared with African Caribbean people who migrated to Britain could be that the experience of the social and environmental factors that lead to mental illness might be more common among non-migrant than migrant members of ethnic minority groups.

The relationship between migration and the prevalence of mental illness among ethnic minority groups is of interest for an additional reason. As described in Chapter 1, it has been suggested that research that uses assessments of mental illness based on western psychiatric practice may fail to identify accurately those from non-western cultures who are ill (Kleinman, 1987; Jadhav, 1996). This could be a consequence of translation difficulties, or a consequence of culturally determined differences in the experience and expression of disease. If either of these possibilities were true, detected rates of mental illness among those who were more acculturated should be higher, in which case those born or educated in Britain and those who spoke English fluently would have higher detected rates of mental illness than those who migrated at an older age or who could not speak English well.

## Using the Fourth National Survey to compare the health of migrant and non-migrant members of ethnic minority communities

A direct test of the health consequences of possible disadvantage associated with migration is, of course, to compare the health of migrants with that of members of ethnic minority groups who were born in Britain. These data will be presented next; however, a number of technical problems occur when a comparison of this sort is made. First, a decision has to be made between what is and what is not a migrant population. Should respondents who migrated in childhood be regarded as migrants, or, because of their exposure to British schooling and a British childhood environment, should they be considered as non-migrants? If we agree with the latter decision, at what age should the cut-off between migrants and non-migrants be made? For the purposes of the comparisons made here, a distinction has been drawn between those who were born in Britain or who migrated below the age of 11 (called non-migrants in the rest of the chapter) and those who migrated aged 11 or older (called migrants in the rest of the chapter). This is somewhat arbitrary and chosen to provide as numerically balanced a sample as possible. However, perhaps because of the small number of respondents affected by such a decision, the results presented are similar to those that are produced if the cut-off is made at the age of 5 or based on country of birth.

The second and perhaps most obvious problem is that the ages of migrant and non-migrant ethnic minority populations in Britain are very different, with little overlap in age groups. For example, in the adult sample of the Fourth National Survey the mean age of Caribbean people born in Britain is 26 (standard deviation = 6) while that of Caribbean people born elsewhere is 50 (standard deviation = 13); the mean age of Indian or African Asian people born in Britain is 22 (standard deviation = 5) while that of Indian or African Asian people born elsewhere is 43 (standard deviation = 14); and the mean age of Pakistani and Bangladeshi people born in Britain is 21 (standard deviation = 4) while that of Pakistani and Bangladeshi people born elsewhere is 39 (standard deviation = 14). This means that only respondents within specific age bands can be used to make the comparison between migrants and non-migrants, and even within these fairly narrow age bands the data need to be age-standardised.

Third, because of differences in when different ethnic groups migrated to Britain, the age bands that are focused on vary from ethnic group to ethnic group. For Caribbean people the age group is 30 to 44, for Indian or African Asian people it is 25 to 39 and for Pakistani or Bangladeshi people it is 20 to 34. This also means that these groups cannot be combined to provide summary figures on migration effects for all ethnic minority people.

Fourth, the need to focus on these relatively young age groups means that the prevalence of ill-health is low among the respondents included for this comparison. Together with the small sample sizes used, this means that comparisons cannot be made for certain illnesses, such as heart disease and diabetes, and for other health assessments differences found will inevitably involve only a small number of respondents. We consequently need to be sensitive to the risk of type II statistical errors, where relevant differences between groups are ignored because they do not meet the criteria for statistical significance (see Blalock, 1985, for a full discussion of this issue).

Finally, differences in detected rates of mental illness between migrants and non-migrants might be a consequence of differences in fluency in English, particularly for those in the South Asian group, and the adequacy of the translation of questions containing complex conceptualisations of health and symptoms. Consequently, this chapter will explore whether rates of mental illness varied among the South Asian groups by English language ability as well as by migration. And, to allow a further exploration of methodological issues, the mental health tables also contain rates for white people who are in the same age groups as the ethnic minority people included here. This will allow a direct comparison between white and ethnic minority rates of mental illness, and whether the differences in the age-standardised relative risks shown in Tables 3.9 and 3.10 apply to both migrants and non-migrants and both those fluent and not fluent in English.

## SELF-ASSESSED GENERAL HEALTH

Table 5.1 is based on responses to the question asking respondents to assess their health on a five-point scale, ranging from excellent to very poor, compared with others of the same age. It shows the percentage of respondents who rated their health as fair, poor or very poor, and that those who migrated aged 11 or older were less likely to have bad health for all ethnic groups. However, differences are only statistically significant for the Caribbean group and are very small for the Pakistani or Bangladeshi group.

**Table 5.1 Reported health compared with others of the same age by age on migration to Britain**

*Cell percentages: age- and gender-standardised*

| | Indian or African Asian | | Pakistani or Bangladeshi | | Caribbean[1] | |
|---|---|---|---|---|---|---|
| | British born or < 11 | 11 or older | British born or < 11 | 11 or older | British born or < 11 | 11 or older |
| Those reporting fair, poor or very poor health | 22.2 | 18.2 | 20.8 | 20.3 | 26.5 | 17.2 |
| *Unweighted base* | *322* | *480* | *316* | *376* | *316* | *111* |

1 p < 0.05.

## SPECIFIC ILLNESSES

Of the five categories of ill-health explored in detail in earlier chapters (heart disease, hypertension, diabetes, respiratory symptoms and accidents) only hypertension and respiratory symptoms occurred frequently enough in the age groups considered here for any meaningful comparisons to be made. Table 5.2 shows responses to the question asking respondents if they had ever had hypertension. Differences for the Indian or African Asian group followed the pattern reported above for self-assessed health, with non-migrants having been more likely than migrants to report hypertension, and are statistically significant. Differences for the other two groups go in the opposite direction, but are not statistically significant.

**Table 5.2    Hypertension by age on migration to Britain**

*Cell percentages: age- and gender-standardised*

|  | Indian or African Asian[1] | | Pakistani or Bangladeshi | | Caribbean | |
|---|---|---|---|---|---|---|
|  | British born or < 11 | 11 or older | British born or < 11 | 11 or older | British born or < 11 | 11 or older |
| Diagnosed hypertension | 3.6 | 1.3 | 2.5 | 4.7 | 8.2 | 9.0 |
| *Unweighted base* | *321* | *479* | *316* | *377* | *314* | *111* |

1 p < 0.05.

**Table 5.3    Respiratory symptoms by age on migration to Britain**

*Cell percentages: age- and gender-standardised*

|  | Indian or African Asian | | Pakistani or Bangladeshi | | Caribbean | |
|---|---|---|---|---|---|---|
|  | British born or < 11 | 11 or older | British born or < 11 | 11 or older | British born or < 11 | 11 or older |
| Wheezing or coughing up phlegm | 13.8 | 8.3 | 8.4 | 7.8 | 21.5 | 11.5 |
| *Unweighted base* | *152* | *241* | *163* | *186* | *160* | *61* |

Half of the ethnic minority sample were asked a series of questions about respiratory symptoms. Table 5.3 shows the rate of positive response to those items most likely to be related to respiratory disease – having either a wheeze or coughing up phlegm for at least three months of the year. Two of the three groups, Indian or African Asian and Caribbean, showed marked differences, with those who migrated to Britain aged 11 or older having had lower rates than others. However, despite the fact that the size of the difference was twofold for the Caribbean group, once again these differences are not statistically significant. The Pakistani or Bangladeshi group showed only small differences between the migrant and non-migrant groups.

## SMOKING

Questions on smoking behaviour were asked of half of the ethnic minority respondents. Consistent with responses to questions on health, Table 5.4 shows that migrants were less likely than non-migrants to have ever smoked for all of the ethnic groups included here. However, these differences are only statistically significant for the Indian or African Asian group, for whom non-migrants are almost twice as likely as migrants to have reported smoking.

**Table 5.4     Smoking by age on migration to Britain**

|  | *Cell percentages: age- and gender-standardised* | | | | | |
|---|---|---|---|---|---|---|
|  | **Indian or African Asian**[1] | | **Pakistani or Bangladeshi** | | **Caribbean** | |
|  | British born or < 11 | 11 or older | British born or < 11 | 11 or older | British born or < 11 | 11 or older |
| Ever smoked | 19.0 | 11.5 | 24.4 | 18.5 | 43.2 | 33.1 |
| *Unweighted base* | *152* | *241* | *163* | *186* | *160* | *61* |

1 p < 0.05.

## NEUROTIC DEPRESSION

Table 5.5 looks at the relationship between age on migration and the estimated weekly prevalence of neurotic depression (which is estimated using the procedure and formula described in Chapter 2) for ethnic minority groups, and also contains the rate for those of the same age in the white group. The table shows a similar effect for the two South Asian groups – migrants had much lower rates of depression than non-migrants. This difference is close to statistical significance for the Indian or African Asian group. For the Caribbean group differences were small, but both migrants and non-migrants reported higher rates than the equivalent white group, as shown for the total Caribbean group in Table 3.9. In contrast to this, for the two South Asian groups the lower than white rate shown in Table 3.9 was only present for those who had migrated to Britain when they were aged 11 or older. Non-migrants in the Pakistani or Bangladeshi group had the same rate as the equivalent white group, while non-migrants in the Indian or African Asian group had a slightly higher rate than the equivalent white group.

Table 5.6 explores the relationship between fluency in English and the estimated prevalence of neurotic depression for the two South Asian groups. The findings mirror those for age on migration. For both the Indian or African Asian group and the Pakistani or Bangladeshi group, those who were fluent in English reported higher rates than those who were not, although the

**Table 5.5    Depression by age on migration to Britain**

|  | Indian or African Asian[1] | | Pakistani or Bangladeshi | | Caribbean | |
|---|---|---|---|---|---|---|
|  | British born or < 11 | 11 or older | British born or < 11 | 11 or older | British born or < 11 | 11 or older |
| Estimated weekly prevalence of depressive neurosis | 5.2 | 1.8 | 3.7 | 1.6 | 7.9 | 6.9 |
| Age-adjusted white rate | | 3.8 | | 3.8 | | 4.3 |
| *Unweighted base* | *152* | *241* | *163* | *186* | *160* | *61* |

*Cell percentages: age- and gender-standardised*

1 p = 0.05.

differences are not statistically significant. Again it is interesting to note that the rate for those who were fluent in English was similar to that for the equivalent white group.

**Table 5.6    Depression by fluency in English**

|  | Indian or African Asian | | Pakistani or Bangladeshi | |
|---|---|---|---|---|
|  | Fluent in English | Not fluent in English | Fluent in English | Not fluent in English |
| Estimated weekly prevalence of depressive neurosis | 3.6 | 2.0 | 3.9 | 1.9 |
| Age-adjusted white rate | | 3.8 | | 3.8 |
| *Unweighted base* | *152* | *241* | *163* | *186* |

*Cell percentages: age- and gender-standardised*

## Non-affective psychosis

Using the formula described in Chapter 2, Table 5.7 shows the estimated annual prevalence of non-affective psychosis among migrant and non-migrant ethnic minority groups. Unlike the findings for rates of admission to hospital (McGovern and Cope, 1987; Harrison et al., 1988), the Caribbean group showed no difference according to age on migration to Britain, with both Caribbean groups having rates about twice that for the equivalent white group. However, the two South Asian groups showed a similar pattern to the findings for neurotic depression, with non-migrants having rates that were twice those of migrants and similar to those for the equivalent white group.

Table 5.8, which shows the relationship between the estimated prevalence of non-affective psychosis and fluency in English for the two South Asian

**Table 5.7    Non-affective psychosis by age on migration to Britain**

*Cell percentages: age- and gender-standardised*

| | Indian or African Asian[1] | | Pakistani or Bangladeshi[1] | | Caribbean | |
|---|---|---|---|---|---|---|
| | British born or < 11 | 11 or older | British born or < 11 | 11 or older | British born or < 11 | 11 or older |
| Estimated annual prevalence of non-affective psychosis | 0.8 | 0.4 | 0.8 | 0.3 | 1.3 | 1.4 |
| Age-adjusted white rate | 0.8 | | 0.8 | | 0.7 | |
| *Unweighted base* | *322* | *480* | *316* | *376* | *316* | *111* |

1 p < 0.01.

groups, also has a similar pattern to that for neurotic depression. Respondents who were fluent in English reported higher rates than those who were not, and for the Pakistani or Bangladeshi group the rate was twice as high and the difference is statistically significant.

**Table 5.8    Non-affective psychosis by fluency in English**

*Cell percentages: age- and gender-standardised*

| | Indian or African Asian | | Pakistani or Bangladeshi[1] | |
|---|---|---|---|---|
| | Fluent in English | Not fluent in English | Fluent in English | Not fluent in English |
| Estimated annual prevalence of non-affective psychosis | 0.6 | 0.4 | 0.8 | 0.4 |
| Age-adjusted white rate | 0.8 | | 0.8 | |
| *Unweighted base* | *322* | *480* | *316* | *376* |

1 p < 0.05.

# UNPACKING MIGRATION AND LANGUAGE EFFECTS FOR MENTAL ILLNESS

Throughout Tables 5.5 to 5.8, fluency in English and age on migration to Britain had similar effects for the two South Asian groups. As these two factors were highly related (very few respondents born or educated in Britain were not fluent in English) this is not surprising. However, in terms of interpreting the findings, they are conceptually very different. If the difference was a result of fluency in English and not age on migration to Britain, the issue could be simply one of inadequate translation. If the difference was one of country of birth and education rather than fluency in English, there would be a stronger case for suggesting that the pattern of findings was a consequence of the problems highlighted by Kleinman (1987) of undertaking cross-cultural psychiatric research. (Of course other explanatory factors, such as socio-economic status, are also related to age on migration and fluency in English, and these may account for the differences shown.)

Table 5.9 explores the inter-relationships between age on migration, fluency in English and mental health (as evidenced by estimated weekly prevalence for depressive neurosis and estimated annual prevalence of non-affective psychosis) for South Asian respondents – who have had to be combined into one broad group because of the small sample size once several factors are considered together. The two right-hand columns consider those who were migrants and show that for this group fluency in English appeared to make no difference and, if anything, was related to a lower rate of illness for the two mental health outcomes. However, the two left-hand columns suggest that there was a relationship between fluency in English and mental illness for those who were non-migrants, with those who were fluent having higher rates for both of the outcomes. A slightly more consistent pattern is suggested by the table for the effect of migration. Comparing the first and third columns shows that among those who were fluent in English, migrants had a much lower rate of mental illness according to the two outcomes considered. And comparing the second and fourth columns shows a similar, although less striking, pattern for those who were not fluent in English.

**Table 5.9    Mental illness, age on migration to Britain and fluency in English for South Asians**

|  | British born or migrated aged under 11 | | Migrated aged 11 or over | |
|  | Fluent in English | Not fluent in English | Fluent in English | Not fluent in English |
| --- | --- | --- | --- | --- |
| *Cell percentages: age- and gender-standardised* | | | | |
| Estimated weekly prevalence of depressive neurosis | 5.1 | 2.3 | 1.3 | 1.9 |
| *Unweighted base* | *245* | *64* | *142* | *271* |
| Estimated annual prevalence of non-affective psychosis | 0.8 | 0.6 | 0.3 | 0.4 |
| *Unweighted base* | *523* | *105* | *276* | *551* |

An alternative way to try and unpack the relative contribution of language and migration effects to the differences shown in earlier tables is to carry out a logistic regression. Here two logistic regression models were tested for the combined South Asian group, each with the main effects of age on migration and fluency in English and the interaction between these as independent variables, but with a different outcome: scoring two or more on the CIS-R; and either being positive on the PSQ or having a diagnosis of psychosis or taking anti-psychotic medication.[2] The findings are presented in Table 5.10, which strongly suggests that the biggest effect was related to age on migration. Fluency in English by itself had little impact on the outcomes (an odds ratio of 1.0 for a variable indicates that it makes no difference to the outcome), although the interaction between fluency and age on migration (i.e. being both fluent and being a non-migrant) did have some effect for the CIS-R (depression) outcome.

**Table 5.10   Logistic regression: age on migration, fluency in English and risk of mental illness for all South Asians combined**

| Variable[1] | Score of two or more on CIS-R<br>Odds ratio | Positive on psychosis screening<br>Odds ratio |
|---|---|---|
| British-born or migrated aged under 11 | 2.3 | 3.2 |
| Fluent in English | 1.0 | 1.5 |
| Interaction term<br>(age on migration x fluency in English) | 1.9 | 0.6 |

1 Age and gender were entered as control variables, but only those of approximately the same age are used to avoid gross age effects (the model remains much the same if all ages are included).

A backward elimination procedure, where the significance of the relationship between dependent and independent variables is used to eliminate from the logistic regression model those variables that do not make an important contribution, was also carried out. The result of this only included age on migration in the models for being positive on psychosis screening. For the CIS-R outcome, migration and the interaction term made similar contributions, as suggested by the full model odds ratios. Overall, then, this suggested that the issue was not one of inadequate translation of the interview materials.

## CONCLUSION

The various assessments of health presented in the tables in this chapter followed the same overall pattern. Although many of the differences between the migrant and non-migrant populations are not statistically significant, in

---

2   Logistic regression depends on having a dichotomous outcome variable (i.e. ill or not ill) rather than one with many categories, which means that the full range of CIS-R or PSQ scores could not be used here, either as outcomes in themselves or to estimate actual rates of depressive or psychotic disorder.

virtually all cases migrants reported better health than non-migrants. In addition, in all cases where the differences *are* statistically significant, migrants reported better health than non-migrants. Taking into account the small size and relatively young age, with consequent low rates of ill-health, of the samples considered (which, as described above, leads to an increased risk of statistical tests missing important differences between groups), the consistency of this evidence across several indicators strongly suggests that for ethnic minority populations in Britain, the health of migrants is as good as that of non-migrants, and is probably better.

Although this conclusion is reasonably clear, its implications for the issues discussed earlier are not so straightforward. This is largely a result of a dependence on cross-sectional survey data. However, data presented by Marmot et al. (1984) suggested that the health of migrants was better than that of those who remained in the country migrated from. This, together with the data presented here, does raise the possibility that selection into migrant groups was at least partly dependent on good health or factors associated with good health, as such an effect would be expected to be diminished for those born in Britain.

The data presented here also indicate that the ethnic inequalities in health, suggested by the findings reported in Chapter 3 and immigrant mortality data published elsewhere (e.g. Marmot et al., 1984), are not the result of environmental factors operating prior to entry to Britain. Such a hypothesis would suggest that those born in Britain, or who migrated at an early age, should be at an advantage compared with the migrant population, which is clearly not the case. Finally, the data also suggest that ethnic inequalities in health cannot be attributed to the stresses and disruptions produced by the process of migration itself. Again, the fact that migrants did not report worse health than non-migrants and, in fact, possibly had better health, is inconsistent with that perspective.

Taken together with the data on smoking, the suggestion that migrants had better health than non-migrants raises an interesting set of further possibilities. Table 5.4 shows that migrants were less likely than non-migrants to have reported that they smoked; consequently, differences in health-related behaviour may have contributed to differences in the health of migrants and non-migrants. Differences in health-related behaviour presumably occur because childhood environment is, in addition to other factors such as ethnic and gender identity, an important influence on the degree to which such practices become culturally acceptable.

In addition, an adverse childhood environment in Britain for non-migrants, compared with the childhood environment of migrants, may also have damaged their adult health more directly. Indeed, there is the possibility that differences in the health of migrants and non-migrants are the result of the non-migrant's greater ongoing exposure to an adverse environment in Britain, rather than a healthy migrant effect. This possibility is strengthened by evidence suggesting that the length of time spent in Britain is directly related to poorer health for migrants from South Asia living in Glasgow (Williams, 1993), with the implication that something about the British environment is damaging their health – although such findings could also be a consequence of positive health selection effects wearing off with time.

In relation to mental illness, for both the Indian or African Asian and the Pakistani or Bangladeshi groups there was a consistent pattern throughout this chapter. Migrants reported lower rates of mental illness than non-migrants for both of the outcomes considered. A similar, although not so strong, pattern emerged when fluency in English was considered, with those who were fluent having higher rates of mental illness than those who were not fluent. However, when age on migration and fluency in English were considered at the same time, it appeared that the main effect was related to the age on migration variable. In fact, given the extent to which attempts were made to overcome translation problems during the fieldwork phase of the Fourth National Survey, with the matching of interviewers and the careful translation of materials, this is perhaps not too surprising. Interestingly, when making a comparison with the rate of mental illness reported by the white group, the tables also showed that the lower rates for the South Asian groups reported in Chapter 3 were not present for those who were fluent in English, or who were born in Britain or migrated under the age of 11.

The interpretation of these mental illness findings is not straightforward. They may reflect a genuine difference in mental health between the migrant and non-migrant South Asian populations. This would not be entirely unexpected; other tables in this chapter show that the physical health of migrants in the South Asian groups is, on the whole, better than that of non-migrants, although the differences were nowhere near as big as those reported for mental health. Elsewhere it has been suggested that the health of migrant populations begins to approximate that of the host population within one or two generations (Syme et al., 1975; Gordon, 1982) and the findings for mental illness follow this pattern. If the findings were a consequence of genuine differences in the health of migrants and non-migrants, two key explanations might be relevant. First, differences could be a consequence of a healthy migrant effect, where the most healthy are selected into the migrant group, an effect that would disappear with subsequent generations. Second, the differences could be a consequence of the negative impact of the British environment on the mental health of ethnic minority people, particularly those who had spent at least part of their early childhood in Britain. Such an effect could be a consequence of cumulative differences in the actual level of disadvantage experienced, or of differences in the interpretation of and response to the disadvantage experienced.

However, we need to consider the possibility that the findings presented in this chapter on mental illness were not a reflection of genuine differences between migrant and non-migrant groups, but a consequence of a measurement artefact related to Kleinman's (1987) category fallacy. The great care that was taken over the translation of materials into different languages and the language matching of interviewers, and the evidence presented from the multivariate analyses (shown in Tables 5.9 and 5.10), suggest that the technical process of translation as such was not an issue here. In fact, when a debriefing of the interviewers used for the follow-up PSE-based study was held, one of the themes raised by the South Asian interviewers from all of the communities in question was the difficulty of translating the concept 'depression' into South Asian languages. Many of the interviewers said that there was no direct equivalent for depression in the relevant languages, that the terms used in the translated interview material were unfamiliar to them, and that interviews in a language other than English took considerably longer than those in English. This clearly raises the possibility that even translated assessments undertaken by ethnically matched interviewers would not be completely effective, and that the concept itself did not translate.

Evidence to support this proposition comes from the tables that showed that age on migration to Britain was strongly related to the possibility of being identified as mentally ill, and that, in addition, age on migration appeared to be more related to this risk than fluency in English. The finding that within the non-migrant group English language ability was related to risk of being identified as mentally ill, while within the migrant group this was not the case (see Table 5.9), also lends strong support to the possibility that the issue is one of cultural distance rather than a direct consequence of the process of migration as discussed above. Those in the combined South Asian group who were born or educated in Britain and were fluent in English would be those who would be expected to be the most acculturated and, consequently, the most likely to be familiar with the western idioms of mental distress used by psychiatric survey instruments. In contrast, it would be expected that both migrant South Asians, and non-migrant South Asians who were not fluent in English, would still have a significant cultural distance from western psychiatry. Overall, the evidence certainly lends strong support to the possibility that the instruments used to assess mental health were, to a certain extent at least, culturally bound and failed to assess adequately the extent of mental illness among the South Asian populations covered by the survey.

Finally it is worth considering the findings on psychotic disorders for the Caribbean group. Chapter 3 suggested that the rates of psychosis among Caribbean people were higher than those for the white group, but not as high as other, treatment-based, research has suggested. It also suggested that these higher rates did not exist for Caribbean men, only being present for Caribbean women, and that there was no evidence for an age or cohort effect among the Caribbean group. This chapter has suggested that the very high treatment rates for psychosis among second-generation African Caribbean people reported elsewhere did not appear in this nationally representative community sample. Here Caribbean people who were born in Britain or who migrated below the age of 11 had almost identical rates of psychosis to those who migrated aged 11 or older, and if the age on migration cut-off was reduced to five years, or to only those born in Britain, the pattern of findings was identical.

# CHAPTER SIX

# Socio-economic effects

## INTRODUCTION

Chapters 3, 4 and 5 of this volume have demonstrated clear ethnic differences in health. Chapter 3 showed that across virtually all of the health dimensions considered, those in the white and Indian or African Asian groups had similar profiles and had better health than that of those in the Caribbean and Pakistani or Bangladeshi groups. The Pakistani or Bangladeshi group had particularly high rates of poor health. In addition, Chapter 4 showed that there were important differences between religious groupings in the Indian or African Asian group, with Muslims, in particular, reporting poorer health than others. These findings clearly indicate that members of ethnic minority groups cannot be considered to be uniformly disadvantaged in respect of their health and, consequently, investigations of the health of ethnic minority people need to consider carefully which ethnic groups they are studying. In addition, these findings suggest a need to consider the extent to which factors that may result in a health disadvantage might vary across ethnic minority groups.

Although there are a number of competing explanations for ethnic differences in health (summarised in Chapter 1 and returned to in the conclusion), given the clearly documented relationship between socio-economic position and health (see, for example, Townsend and Davidson, 1982; Blaxter, 1987 and 1990; Davey Smith et al., 1990a; Benzeval et al., 1995; Independent Inquiry into Inequalities in Health, 1998) and the relatively deprived position of many ethnic minority groups (Modood et al., 1997), it seems that any exploration of ethnic differences in health needs to consider socio-economic effects seriously. Table 6.1 looks at some indicators of socio-economic position using data from the Fourth National Survey. It shows the occupational class distributions of different ethnic minority groups, together with their unemployment rates and the number that live in poor quality housing.

Across all three of these dimensions of socio-economic position, the Indian or African Asian group compares favourably with the white group. Those in the Caribbean and Pakistani or Bangladeshi groups are clearly worse off than white and Indian or African Asian people, with Pakistani or Bangladeshi people the most disadvantaged. The fact that the inequalities in socio-economic position across ethnic groups follow the general pattern for health adds weight to the suggestion that this may, on prima facie grounds, be a fruitful avenue to explore. However, the role that differences in socio-economic position may play in determining ethnic inequalities in health is the subject of considerable debate, with some claiming that it makes a minimal or no contribution to ethnic inequalities in health (Wild and McKeigue, 1997), others suggesting that even if it does contribute, the cultural and genetic elements of ethnicity must also play a role (Smaje, 1996), and others arguing that ethnic inequalities in health are predominantly determined by socio-economic inequalities (Navarro, 1990; Sheldon and Parker, 1992).

**Table 6.1    Ethnic differences in socio-economic position**

*Cell percentages*

|  | White | Indian or African Asian | Pakistani or Bangladeshi | Caribbean |
|---|---|---|---|---|
| **Registrar General's class** |  |  |  |  |
| I/II | 35 | 32 | 17 | 22 |
| IIIn | 15 | 21 | 16 | 18 |
| IIIm | 31 | 22 | 32 | 30 |
| IV/V | 20 | 26 | 35 | 30 |
| *Unweighted base* | *2239* | *1772* | *1262* | *1057* |
| **Economically active who are unemployed** | 11 | 15 | 39 | 24 |
| *Unweighted base* | *1603* | *1238* | *812* | *814* |
| **Lacking one or more basic housing amenities**[1] | 16 | 16 | 37 | 17 |
| *Unweighted base* | *2867* | *2001* | *1776* | *1205* |

1 This includes exclusive use of bath or shower; bathroom; inside toilet; kitchen; hot water from a tap; and central heating.

Empirical attempts to explore the relationship between socio-economic position, ethnicity and health have generally not lent support to the perspective that socio-economic inequalities play a role. The negative evidence of Marmot et al.'s (1984) immigrant mortality study, which was published in the context of the Black report (Townsend and Davidson, 1982), has already been described (see Chapter 1). Since then, it took until 1997 for socio-economic position to regain a prominent position in published national data exploring the relationship between country of birth and mortality rates in Britain (Harding and Maxwell, 1997). This analysis was conducted in the context of the British inequalities in health decennial supplement (Drever and Whitehead, 1997) and again used census and death certificate data to explore mortality rates by country of birth. In contrast to Marmot et al.'s (1984) findings, Harding and Maxwell (1997) showed clear socio-economic gradients in mortality rates for migrant groups. Despite this, as for the earlier analysis, they found that controlling for occupational class made no contribution to the differences between different country of birth groups. This led Harding and Maxwell to conclude that:

> Among the non-white ethnic groups, the relationship between social class and mortality is becoming apparent in the 1990s for groups who have settled here for some time. Our overall conclusion, however, supports the earlier ones that social class is not an adequate explanation for the patterns of excess mortality observed (Harding and Maxwell 1997: 120).

So, although the most recent evidence from immigrant mortality studies suggests that there are socio-economic gradients in health for all ethnic groups, they also continue to suggest that differences in socio-economic position do not contribute to ethnic inequalities in health in Britain.

Other studies have also failed to find a relationship between socio-economic position and health within certain ethnic groups for specific illnesses (e.g. Clarke et al., 1988), and they have also found that standardising for socio-economic position across ethnic groups did not greatly diminish the relationship between ethnicity and health, even if within ethnic groups there was an association between socio-economic position and health (e.g. Fenton et al., 1995; Smaje, 1995a). (However, Ahmad et al., 1989, were able to show that once unemployment had been controlled for, South Asian men living in Bradford had better, rather than worse, health than their white counterparts.)

It is possible that both the within- and between-group negative findings for the relationship between socio-economic position and health are a result of the use of socio-economic indicators that inadequately reflect the position of ethnic minority groups. In fact, there has been an increasing recognition of the limitations of traditional class groupings, which are far from internally homogeneous. A number of studies have drawn attention to inequalities in income levels and death rates among the occupations that comprise each occupational class (e.g. Davey Smith et al., 1990b). And within an occupational group, ethnic minorities may be more likely to be found in lower or less prestigious occupational grades, to have poorer job security, to endure more stressful working conditions and to be more likely to work unsocial hours. Bartley's (1994) work, which demonstrates that those who have insecure work, or who have been obliged to take on low-status jobs, have a similar risk of poor health to the unemployed, illustrates the significance of this.

Alternative measures of material circumstances, which are easy to collect and apparently universally applicable, have also been used as socio-economic indicators in epidemiological work – typically housing tenure and car ownership.

An increasing number of studies report large inequalities in health associated with these measures of socio-economic position (e.g. Townsend et al., 1988). However, advocates of the use of such measures have often failed to consider how ethnicity interacts with them. For example, although the proportion of home owners is higher in most South Asian groups than among whites, the quality of their accommodation tends to be poorer (Brown, 1984; Modood et al., 1997). In fact, the most disadvantaged, who undoubtably include a large proportion of certain ethnic minority groups, probably suffer disproportionately from the cumulative impact of different forms of deprivation, an effect which cannot be identified by a one-dimensional indicator of socio-economic position.

## THE IMPACT OF OCCUPATIONAL CLASS AND TENURE WITHIN ETHNIC GROUPS

Clearly these issues require detailed consideration, and the data available from the Fourth National Survey provide a unique opportunity to do this. To begin with, for each of the ethnic groups the relationship between two standard indicators of socio-economic position – occupational class and tenure – and health assessments will be explored. For tenure, a simple distinction between owner-occupiers and renters will be made. For occupational class, a distinction will be drawn between households that are manual and those that are non-manual, according to the Registrar General's criteria,[1] and, in addition to this, a third group of respondents from households containing no full-time worker will be included (for reasons described shortly, respondents aged 65 or older have not been included in any of the analyses presented in this chapter). Once these issues have been explored, the limitations of these standard indicators of socio-economic position for making comparisons across ethnic groups will be examined, and a possible way forward will be developed. This will show how controlling for socio-economic position in different ways alters our understanding of the factors underlying ethnic inequalities in health.

The health indicators used here reflect the broad topics covered in earlier chapters and include self-assessed health compared with others of the same age; diagnosed heart disease; diagnosed heart disease or severe chest pain; hypertension; diabetes; symptoms suggestive of respiratory disease; smoking; neurotic depression; and non-affective psychosis.

Once again the data presented in this chapter have been age- and gender-standardised to allow for immediate comparisons across both socio-economic and ethnic groups. This means that, because of small numbers in particular weighting cells, the 65 and older age group have not been included in the data

---

1    Class was assigned using the head of the household's occupation. Where it was not clear which household member was the head of the household (e.g. where there was more than one working adult), class was allocated on the basis of gender (with men's occupations being used in preference to women's) and age (e.g. a father's occupations being used in preference to a son's).

presented in this chapter, which means that they are not directly comparable with those shown in earlier chapters.

## Self-assessed general health

Respondents were asked to rate their health in comparison with others of the same age on a five-point scale ranging from very poor to very good. The first part of Table 6.2 shows the percentage of respondents in each ethnic group who said that they had fair, poor or very poor health by whether they lived in a household that had no full-time worker, or was manual or non-manual. It shows a very clear and significant relationship between this indicator of general health and socio-economic position for all ethnic groups. Interestingly, the difference between individuals in manual and non-manual households appears to be more marked for ethnic minority than white respondents.

**Table 6.2    Fair, poor, or very poor reported health compared with others of the same age by socio-economic position**

|  | | *Cell percentages: age- and gender-standardised* | | |
|---|---|---|---|---|
|  | White[1] | Indian or African Asian[2] | Pakistani or Bangladeshi[3] | Caribbean[4] |
| **Occupational class** | | | | |
| Non-manual | 21.5 | 19.9 | 30.2 | 25.0 |
| Manual | 22.6 | 27.4 | 35.1 | 29.4 |
| No full-time worker in household | 36.7 | 33.9 | 44.1 | 38.2 |
| *Unweighted base* | *2110* | *1782* | *1592* | *1060* |
| **Tenure** | | | | |
| Owner-occupier | 22.6 | 24.4 | 34.7 | 26.6 |
| Tenant | 34.5 | 33.7 | 45.0 | 40.0 |
| *Unweighted base* | *2173* | *1848* | *1692* | *1077* |

1 $p < 0.01$ for both occupational class and tenure.
2 $p < 0.01$ for both occupational class and tenure.
3 $p < 0.01$ for both occupational class and tenure.
4 $p < 0.01$ for both occupational class and tenure.

The second part of Table 6.2 looks at how responses to the same question varied between those who rented their accommodation and those who owned it. Again there is a clear and significant relationship: those who owned their homes were less likely than those who rented to report fair or worse health for all of the ethnic groups.

*Ethnicity, Class and Health*

## Heart disease

Table 6.3 shows the percentage of respondents who reported a diagnosis of angina or heart attack within each ethnic grouping by occupational class and tenure. It shows a similar pattern to that for self-assessed general health, although not quite as clear. In the first half of Table 6.3, the expected relationship between occupational class and diagnosed heart disease is present for the Indian or African Asian and the Pakistani or Bangladeshi groups. However, for the Caribbean and white groups, people in non-manual households were more likely to report a diagnosis of heart disease than those in manual households.

**Table 6.3    Diagnosed angina or heart attack[1] by socio-economic position**

*Cell percentages: age- and gender-standardised*

|  | White | Indian or African Asian[2] | Pakistani or Bangladeshi[3] | Caribbean |
|---|---|---|---|---|
| **Occupational class** | | | | |
| Non-manual | 3.0 | 1.4 | 2.8 | 3.3 |
| Manual | 2.7 | 3.2 | 6.1 | 2.7 |
| No full-time worker in household | 3.9 | 4.3 | 5.4 | 4.0 |
| *Unweighted base* | *2110* | *1783* | *1593* | *1060* |
| **Tenure** | | | | |
| Owner-occupier | 3.0 | 2.5 | 5.2 | 2.7 |
| Tenant | 4.1 | 3.5 | 5.2 | 3.8 |
| *Unweighted base* | *2173* | *1849* | *1694* | *1077* |

1 In addition to 'heart attack', the question wording added 'including a heart murmur, a damaged heart or a rapid heart'.
2 p < 0.01 for occupational class.
3 p < 0.05 for occupational class.

The second part of Table 6.3 shows that home owners were less likely to report diagnosed heart disease than renters in each of the ethnic groups except the Pakistani or Bangladeshi group, although none of the differences shown is statistically significant.

Respondents aged 40 or more were also asked questions about the experience of chest pain. The first part of Table 6.4 shows that for all of the ethnic groups there was the expected relationship between occupational class and either having a diagnosis of heart disease or experiencing severe chest pain, although for the Pakistani or Bangladeshi group those in households without a full-time worker were less likely than those in manual households to have reported one of these indicators of heart disease.

The second part of Table 6.4 confirms this overall impression. Home owners were less likely than those who rent to report either a diagnosis of heart disease or severe chest pain for all of the ethnic groups except the Pakistani or Bangladeshi group, although differences for the Caribbean group were small.

**Table 6.4    Diagnosed heart disease[1] or severe chest pain by socio-economic position[2]**

|  | | | *Cell percentages: age- and gender-standardised* | |
|  | White[3] | Indian or African Asian[4] | Pakistani or Bangladeshi[5] | Caribbean |
|---|---|---|---|---|
| **Occupational class** | | | | |
| Non-manual | 8.3 | 6.9 | 9.8 | 8.7 |
| Manual | 10.6 | 11.3 | 27.1 | 11.3 |
| No full-time worker in household | 19.4 | 17.2 | 23.6 | 12.3 |
| *Unweighted base* | *919* | *654* | *475* | *369* |
| **Tenure** | | | | |
| Owner-occupier | 10.8 | 10.7 | 23.3 | 11.0 |
| Tenant | 15.5 | 18.2 | 21.1 | 11.5 |
| *Unweighted base* | *939* | *680* | *514* | *374* |

1 In addition to 'heart attack', the question wording added 'including a heart murmur, a damaged heart or a rapid heart'.
2 Only those aged 40 or older are included here.
3 $p < 0.05$ for tenure.
4 $p < 0.01$ for occupational class and $p = 0.051$ for tenure.
5 $p < 0.05$ for occupational class.

## Hypertension

Table 6.5 shows the relationship between socio-economic position and reporting a diagnosis of hypertension. Although the first part of the table shows that, for Indian or African Asian and white people, those in households with no full-time worker were less likely than those in manual households to report such a diagnosis, and there was no difference between manual and non-manual Caribbean people, overall the expected inverse relationship between occupational class and a diagnosis of hypertension is present.

The relationship between socio-economic position and likelihood to have reported a diagnosis of hypertension for all ethnic groups is confirmed in the second part of Table 6.5, although the difference within the Caribbean group was again not statistically significant.

**Table 6.5    Diagnosed hypertension by socio-economic position**

| | White[1] | Indian or African Asian[2] | Pakistani or Bangladeshi[3] | Caribbean |
|---|---|---|---|---|
| | | *Cell percentages: age- and gender-standardised* | | |
| **Occupational class** | | | | |
| Non-manual | 8.0 | 4.3 | 5.8 | 14.7 |
| Manual | 11.6 | 9.0 | 9.5 | 14.8 |
| No full-time worker in household | 10.6 | 7.9 | 11.3 | 17.7 |
| *Unweighted base* | *2111* | *1780* | *1591* | *1055* |
| **Tenure** | | | | |
| Owner-occupier | 9.5 | 6.2 | 8.9 | 13.9 |
| Tenant | 12.6 | 9.4 | 12.0 | 16.6 |
| *Unweighted base* | *2173* | *1846* | *1692* | *1072* |

1 p < 0.05 for both occupational class and tenure.
2 p < 0.01 for occupational class and p < 0.05 for tenure.
3 p < 0.05 for both occupational class and tenure.

## Diabetes

Table 6.6 shows the relationship between having reported a diagnosis of diabetes and occupational class and tenure. Although the relationship is not entirely consistent, the first part of the table does suggest that there is a relationship between occupational class and such a diagnosis for all ethnic groups except, possibly, Caribbean people. This is confirmed in the tenure part of the table, which shows that for all except the Pakistani or Bangladeshi group, home owners were less likely than renters to report a diagnosis of diabetes.

## Respiratory disease

Half of the ethnic minority and all of the white respondents were asked a number of questions about symptoms relating to respiratory disease. Table 6.7 shows the percentage of respondents who reported that either they had a wheeze or that they had coughed up phlegm for at least three months of the year, by occupational class and tenure. Again, the table suggests a strong and significant relationship between socio-economic position and respiratory symptoms, although it is not completely consistent in the occupational class part of the table.

## Table 6.6 Diagnosed diabetes by socio-economic position

*Cell percentages: age- and gender-standardised*

| | White[1] | Indian or African Asian[2] | Pakistani or Bangladeshi | Caribbean[3] |
|---|---|---|---|---|
| **Occupational class** | | | | |
| Non-manual | 1.1 | 2.8 | 6.4 | 4.1 |
| Manual | 1.1 | 3.5 | 8.3 | 3.3 |
| No full-time worker in household | 2.1 | 7.1 | 7.6 | 4.5 |
| *Unweighted base* | *2111* | *1785* | *1593* | *1059* |
| **Tenure** | | | | |
| Owner-occupier | 1.1 | 3.7 | 7.6 | 2.5 |
| Tenant | 2.7 | 5.9 | 6.9 | 6.0 |
| *Unweighted base* | *2174* | *1851* | *1694* | *1076* |

1 p < 0.01 for tenure.
2 p < 0.01 for occupational class.
3 p < 0.01 for tenure.

## Table 6.7 Wheezing or coughing up phlegm by socio-economic position

*Cell percentages: age- and gender-standardised*

| | White[1] | Indian or African Asian[2] | Pakistani or Bangladeshi[3] | Caribbean[4] |
|---|---|---|---|---|
| **Occupational class** | | | | |
| Non-manual | 23.3 | 12.8 | 13.1 | 16.3 |
| Manual | 23.2 | 12.7 | 12.0 | 27.6 |
| No full-time worker in household | 35.1 | 17.5 | 20.0 | 26.2 |
| *Unweighted base* | *2113* | *872* | *780* | *534* |
| **Tenure** | | | | |
| Owner-occupier | 24.3 | 11.9 | 15.9 | 20.8 |
| Tenant | 31.8 | 23.7 | 20.5 | 26.6 |
| *Unweighted base* | *2176* | *910* | *836* | *546* |

1 p < 0.01 for both occupational class and tenure.
2 p < 0.01 for tenure.
3 p < 0.05 for occupational class.
4 p < 0.05 for occupational class.

# Smoking

Table 6.8 shows the relationship between current regular smoking and occupational class and tenure for each ethnic group. The first part of the table shows that those with no full-time worker in the home were more likely than those in manual homes to smoke, and that those in non-manual homes were the least likely to smoke, although the relationship is not entirely consistent for the two South Asian groups.

**Table 6.8    Currently smoke regularly[1] by socio-economic position**

|  | | | *Cell percentages: age- and gender-standardised* |
|---|---|---|---|
|  | White[2] | Indian or African Asian[3] | Pakistani or Bangladeshi[4] | Caribbean[5] |
| **Occupational class** | | | | |
| Non-manual | 21.3 | 8.8 | 15.8 | 24.3 |
| Manual | 33.2 | 8.1 | 18.3 | 30.2 |
| No full-time worker in household | 46.2 | 18.7 | 18.1 | 39.4 |
| *Unweighted base* | *2113* | *872* | *780* | *534* |
| **Tenure** | | | | |
| Owner-occupier | 23.9 | 7.8 | 14.1 | 21.1 |
| Tenant | 45.1 | 18.3 | 24.5 | 40.9 |
| *Unweighted base* | *2176* | *910* | *836* | *546* |

1 Regular is more than one a day.
2 $p < 0.01$ for both occupational class and tenure.
3 $p < 0.01$ for both occupational class and tenure.
4 $p < 0.01$ for tenure.
5 $p < 0.01$ for both occupational class and tenure.

This finding is confirmed in the second part of Table 6.8, which shows that home owners were much less likely to be smokers than renters for all of the ethnic groups.

# Neurotic depression

Table 6.9 shows the relationship between estimated weekly prevalence of depression and socio-economic position. The first part of the table shows that for three of the ethnic groups, white, Indian or African Asian and Caribbean, there was a reasonably clear relationship. Overall, those in non-manual households had the lowest rate of depression and those in households with no full-time worker had the highest rate, although there was no difference between the manual and non-manual groups for Caribbean people. For the

Pakistani or Bangladeshi group there did not appear to be any clear relationship between occupational class and the risk of having depression.

**Table 6.9    Estimated weekly prevalence of depressive neurosis by socio-economic position**

|  | *Cell percentages: age- and gender-standardised* | | | |
| --- | --- | --- | --- | --- |
|  | White[1] | Indian or African Asian[2] | Pakistani or Bangladeshi | Caribbean |
| **Occupational class** | | | | |
| Non-manual | 2.6 | 2.0 | 3.3 | 5.8 |
| Manual | 4.1 | 3.1 | 2.6 | 5.4 |
| No full-time worker in household | 6.8 | 5.3 | 3.2 | 7.7 |
| *Unweighted base* | *2107* | *871* | *780* | *533* |
| **Tenure** | | | | |
| Owner-occupier | 3.4 | 2.1 | 3.0 | 4.2 |
| Tenant | 5.6 | 7.8 | 2.7 | 7.4 |
| *Unweighted base* | *2170* | *909* | *836* | *545* |

1 $p < 0.01$ for occupational class and $p < 0.05$ for tenure.
2 $p < 0.05$ for occupational class and $p < 0.01$ for tenure.

The second part of the table confirms this impression. For three of the ethnic groups, white, Caribbean and Indian or African Asian, there was a clear relationship between tenure and risk of depression, while for those in the Pakistani or Bangladeshi group there appeared to be no relationship.

# Non-affective psychosis

Differences in the estimated annual prevalence of non-affective psychosis by socio-economic position and ethnic group are shown in Table 6.10.

For the white group the table shows that there was a strong and significant inverse relationship with both occupational class and tenure. A similar, but not so strong, pattern was also present for the Indian or African Asian group, while, once again, there was no clear relationship for the Pakistani or Bangladeshi group. For the Caribbean group, although differences were not statistically significant, as expected those from households with no full-time worker had the highest rates of psychosis – the estimated annual prevalence of non-affective psychosis was almost 2 per cent for this group – and tenants had higher rates than owner-occupiers. However, unexpectedly, those in non-manual households appeared to have higher rates than those from manual households.

**Table 6.10  Estimated annual prevalence of non-affective psychosis by socio-economic position**

| | White[1] | Indian or African Asian[2] | Pakistani or Bangladeshi | Caribbean |
|---|---|---|---|---|
| | | | *Cell percentages: age- and gender-standardised* | |
| **Occupational class** | | | | |
| Non-manual | 0.4 | 0.5 | 0.6 | 1.5 |
| Manual | 0.8 | 0.5 | 0.4 | 1.1 |
| No full-time worker in household | 1.7 | 1.1 | 0.6 | 1.9 |
| *Unweighted base* | *2107* | *1783* | *1595* | *1059* |
| **Tenure** | | | | |
| Owner-occupier | 0.7 | 0.5 | 0.6 | 1.2 |
| Tenant | 1.2 | 1.5 | 0.5 | 1.6 |
| *Unweighted base* | *2170* | *1849* | *1696* | *1077* |

1 p < 0.01 for occupational class.
2 p = 0.053 for tenure.

## Summary

The data presented in Tables 6.2 to 6.10 showed a reasonably clear and consistent relationship between socio-economic position and health for all of the main health indicators used in this survey and for each of the ethnic groups covered. This is much as might be expected from studies of the general population, and, like such studies, tenure on the whole had a stronger and more consistent relationship with health outcomes than a combined indicator of Registrar General's class and unemployment (see, for example, Haynes 1991). Interestingly, however, the opposite was the case for the Pakistani or Bangladeshi group, for whom the occupational class measure seemed to have a stronger relationship with the health outcomes than tenure. The Pakistani or Bangladeshi group also did not show socio-economic gradients for the mental health outcomes, even though there was a clear and inverse relationship for the white and Indian or African Asian groups for both outcomes and both assessments of socio-economic position. Overall, for the white, Indian or African Asian and Caribbean groups there was the expected inverse relationship between socio-economic status and mental health for both depression and psychosis. However, there was one interesting exception to this among the Caribbean group – while those from households with no full-time worker had the expected highest rate of mental illness, those from non-manual households had higher rates than those from manual households.

## ADJUSTING FOR SOCIO-ECONOMIC DIFFERENCES BETWEEN ETHNIC GROUPS

Given that there is such a strong relationship between socio-economic position and health within particular ethnic groups, and there are important differences in the socio-economic positions of different ethnic groups (as illustrated in Table 6.1), it would seem to make sense to explore how far ethnic differences in health remain once socio-economic inequalities between ethnic groups had been adjusted for. This is the strategy adopted in the analysis of immigrant mortality rates by both Marmot et al. (1984) and Harding and Maxwell (1997), but, as previously described, they found that once they had standardised for occupational class, ethnic differences in health remained more or less unchanged. A similar impression might be formed from the data presented in Tables 6.2 to 6.10. For example, in Table 6.2 within each occupational class group and each tenure group Pakistani or Bangladeshi people were more likely than white people to report fair, poor, or very poor health. Indeed, if all of the tables are looked at in this way, it seems that we should conclude that while there are important socio-economic effects *within* ethnic groups, differences *between* ethnic groups remain once these have been accounted for. That is, socio-economic factors do not appear to explain ethnic differences in health.

However, some thought has to be given to how adequate variables such as occupational class and tenure are for controlling out socio-economic effects when exploring ethnic inequalities in health. In effect, we have to ask ourselves whether individuals from different ethnic groups, but within the same broad socio-economic band – such as non-manual or owner-occupier – are really in an equivalent socio-economic position. It certainly seems possible that within these broad bands ethnic minority people will be worse off than white people. This, then, suggests that the process of standardising for socio-economic position when making comparisons across ethnic groups is not as straightforward as it might at first sight seem. As Kaufman et al. (1997 and 1998) point out, the process of standardisation is effectively an attempt to deal with the non-random nature of differences in explanatory factors between samples used in cross-sectional studies – controlling for all relevant 'extraneous' explanatory factors introduces the appearance of randomisation. But, given the potential non-equivalence of socio-economic measures across ethnic groups, attempting to introduce randomisation into cross-sectional studies by adding socio-economic 'controls' has a number of problems. Kaufman et al. summarise these in the following way:

> When considering socio-economic exposures and making comparisons between racial/ethnic groups the material, behavioral, and psychological circumstances of diverse socio-economic and racial/ethnic groups are distinct on so many dimensions that no realistic adjustment can plausibly simulate randomization (Kaufman et al., 1998:147).

This issue is explored empirically for the Fourth National Survey sample in Table 6.11.

The first part of Table 6.11 shows the mean equivalised household income for individuals within particular classes by ethnic group. This statistic needs to be treated with some caution for a number of reasons. First, a large number of individuals did not reply to the question asking about household income. Second, although the calculation is weighted to take into account the number of adults and children in the household, it is based on income bands rather than actual incomes. In order to perform the calculations, the mid-point of each band has been taken, but this inevitably produces some inaccuracy, particularly if members of different ethnic groups are differentially located within the bands used. Nevertheless, the table does show that Caribbean and Indian or African Asian people appear to have similar locations within each occupational class, while white people were better off than they were, and Pakistani or Bangladeshi people were worse off than they were. Indeed, comparing the white and Pakistani or Bangladeshi groups shows that within each occupational class band, those in the Pakistani or Bangladeshi group had on average half the white income, and class I or II Pakistani or Bangladeshi people had an equivalent average income to class IV or V white people. Despite the element of inaccuracy in the calculation of the income figure, the consistency of the pattern in each occupational class suggests that standardising for Registrar General's class is a far from adequate method of dealing with socio-economic effects for comparisons across ethnic groups.

The second part of the table shows the median length of unemployment for those who were currently unemployed at interview. It again shows diverse patterns across ethnic groups, with those in the white and Indian or African Asian groups having been unemployed for a considerably shorter period than those in the Caribbean and Pakistani or Bangladeshi groups. Here it is worth noting that Bartley et al. (1996) clearly showed that length of unemployment, rather than unemployment per se, was an important determinant of health.

The third part of Table 6.11 gives an indication of the quality of housing occupied by owners and renters for different ethnic groups. It shows the percentage of respondents who reported that their household did not have sole access to certain amenities: a bath or shower; a bathroom; an inside toilet; a kitchen; hot water from a tap; and central heating. Again the table shows interesting differences across ethnic groups. For both owners and renters, the white, Caribbean and Indian or African Asian groups show a similar pattern, while those in the Pakistani or Bangladeshi group are far more likely to be lacking exclusive use of such an amenity than any other group in both the owner and the renter categories. In addition, while owners appear to have better housing than renters for the white, Caribbean and Indian or African Asian groups, this is not the case for the Pakistani or Bangladeshi group. This, of course, suggests that tenure may not only be an inadequate means of controlling for socio-economic position when making comparisons across ethnic groups, but also that tenure is an inadequate reflection of socio-

**Table 6.11    Ethnic variations in socio-economic position within socio-economic bands**

|  | White | Indian or African Asian | Pakistani or Bangladeshi | Caribbean |
|---|---|---|---|---|
| **Mean income by Registrar General's class pounds**[1] |  |  |  |  |
| I/II | 250 | 210 | 125 | 210 |
| IIIn | 185 | 135 | 95 | 145 |
| IIIm | 160 | 120 | 70 | 145 |
| IV/V | 130 | 110 | 65 | 120 |
| *Unweighted base* | *1894* | *1142* | *969* | *869* |
| **Median duration of unemployment months** | 7 | 12 | 24 | 21 |
| *Unweighted base* | *128* | *91* | *166* | *91* |
| **Per cent lacking one or more basic housing amenities**[2] |  |  |  |  |
| Owner-occupiers | 11 | 14 | 38 | 12 |
| Renters | 27 | 28 | 37 | 23 |
| *Unweighted base* | *2867* | *2001* | *1776* | *1205* |

1 Based on bands of equivalised household income. The mean point of each band is used to make this calculation, which is rounded to the nearest 5.
2 This includes exclusive use of bath or shower; bathroom; inside toilet; kitchen; hot water from a tap; and central heating.

economic position within the Pakistani or Bangladeshi group. And this might explain why tenure was less likely to be associated with health status for Pakistani or Bangladeshi people than those in the other ethnic groups.

The overall conclusion to be drawn from Table 6.11 is that, while these indicators of socio-economic position might have some use for making comparisons within ethnic groups (for example the first part of the table shows that equivalised household income decreases with occupational class for each ethnic group), they are of little use for 'controlling out' the impact of socio-economic position when attempting to reveal the extent of a 'non-socio-economic' ethnic/race effect. And similar findings have been reported in the US (Lillie-Blanton and Laveist, 1994; Williams et al., 1994). This leads to two related problems with approaches that attempt to adjust for socio-economic effects when making comparisons across ethnic groups. The first of these is that if socio-economic position is simply regarded as a confounding factor that needs to be controlled out to reveal the 'true' relationship between ethnicity and health, data will be presented and interpreted once controls have been applied. This will result in the impact of socio-economic factors actually becoming obscured and their explanatory role lost.

The second is that the presentation of 'standardised' data allows the problems with such data, illustrated by Table 6.11, to be ignored, leaving both the author and reader to assume that all that is left is an 'ethnic/race' effect, be that cultural or genetic/biological. Here it is important to remember that not only do such socio-economic indicators deal inadequately with these effects for cross-group comparisons, they also do not account for other forms of disadvantage that might play some role in ethnic inequalities in health, such as those related to geographical location and the direct effects of racism and discrimination, both described in Chapter 1.

Nevertheless, if these cautions are considered, there are some benefits in attempting to control for socio-economic effects. In particular, if controlling for socio-economic effects alters the pattern of ethnic inequalities in health, despite the limitations of the indicators used, we can conclude that at least a part of the differences we have uncovered is a result of such an effect. To do this we need to consider carefully which indicators to use in the process of standardisation for socio-economic position. There are a number of alternatives to those typically used in epidemiological research, including income. However, there are a number of drawbacks associated with income in the Fourth National Survey, most importantly that there was a sufficiently large number of respondents who did not answer the relevant question and this non-response varied by both ethnic group and occupational class. This makes it less useful than it at first appears for anything other than a cross-check.

Instead, making use of the extensive information this survey collected on the circumstances of its respondents, an index of 'Standard of Living' will be used in addition to occupational class and tenure for the process of standardisation. This index, like the other indicators of socio-economic position used, is household-based, using information on overcrowding of the accommodation; the presence of basic household amenities; the number of consumer durables the household has; and the number of cars the household has access to. The index has three mutually exclusive points to it, poor, medium and good, that are inevitably broad, but have been selected both because of their face validity and because they each contain a reasonably large sample size for each ethnic group. Simplifying the index slightly, the 'poor' group consists of those with any of the following:

- overcrowded accommodation (one or more people per room); or
- lacking sole access to one or more amenity (out of a bath or shower; a bathroom; an inside toilet; a kitchen; hot water from a tap; and central heating); or
- few consumer durables (less than four of a telephone; television; video; fridge; freezer; washing machine; tumble-drier; dishwasher; microwave; CD-player; and personal computer).

The 'good' group consists of those with *all* of the following:

- less than 0.75 people per room; and
- sole access to all of the basic amenities listed above; and
- many of the consumer durables listed above (nine or more, or five or more and two cars).

The relationship between this index and ethnic group is shown in Table 6.12. This shows that the white group was the best off, followed closely by the Indian or African Asian group. The Caribbean group was clearly worse off than either of these two, but the Pakistani or Bangladeshi group was by far the worst off.

## Table 6.12   Standard of living

|  | | | | *Column percentages* |
| --- | --- | --- | --- | --- |
|  | White | Indian or African Asian | Pakistani or Bangladeshi | Caribbean |
| **Standard of living** | | | | |
| Good | 43 | 34 | 9 | 23 |
| Medium | 49 | 52 | 41 | 63 |
| Poor | 8 | 14 | 50 | 14 |
| *Unweighted base* | *2865* | *1996* | *1776* | *1205* |

The small percentage of people in the poor band for the white group and the good band for the Pakistani or Bangladeshi group shows why it was necessary for the three bands that make up this index to be relatively broad. However, this raises the possibility that once again different ethnic groups have different locations within a particular band. This is explored in Table 6.13, which looks at the equivalised household income for each band by ethnic group. As expected, within ethnic groups there was a clear relationship between income and the standard of living index. Comparisons across ethnic groups show that the white, Caribbean and Indian or African Asian groups were similar, except for the relatively low average income for Indian or African Asian people in the medium group. However, within each band the Pakistani or Bangladeshi group had a lower average income than others. This suggests that the standard of living index still does not adequately control for socio-economic position and reinforces Kaufman et al.'s (1998) point. Nevertheless, a comparison between the data presented in Table 6.11 and those in Table 6.13 shows that the ratio between the incomes of the Pakistani or Bangladeshi and white groups for each socio-economic band is smaller in the latter table, suggesting that it should be an improvement over the other indicators of socio-economic position, which are, if anything, even cruder than Registrar General's class.

The remainder of this chapter will show how standardising for the three indicators of socio-economic position influences the ethnic patterning of health reported in Chapter 3. The data will be presented as relative risk scores in comparison with the white group, with 95 per cent confidence limits shown in brackets.

**Table 6.13    Ethnic differences in income by standard of living**

|  | White | Indian or African Asian | Pakistani or Bangladeshi | Caribbean |
|---|---|---|---|---|
| **Mean income by standard of living (£)[1]** |  |  |  |  |
| Good | 225 | 210 | 155 | 195 |
| Medium | 145 | 115 | 80 | 140 |
| Poor | 105 | 95 | 65 | 100 |
| | | | | |
| *Unweighted base* | *2410* | *1283* | *1327* | *991* |

1 Based on bands of equivalised household income. The mean point of each band is used to make this calculation, which is rounded to the nearest 5.

As the data have been standardised according to age, gender and the socio-economic indicator in question and as there were too few respondents in particular categories above the age of 65 for them to be included, these older respondents have been dropped from the tables. This includes the data that are presented here in just age- and gender-standardised form, which means the age- and gender-standardised relative risks presented here are not identical to those shown in Chapter 3, which include all age groups, although they are similar.

## General health

Table 6.14 looks at the effect of various forms of standardisation on the relative risk compared with white people for the respondent to have described his or her health as fair, poor, or very poor. The most striking finding shown in the table is that standardising for occupational class or tenure makes no difference to the relative risk for the Pakistani or Bangladeshi group. However, controlling for standard of living reduces the difference between the Pakistani or Bangladeshi and white groups to one that is only just statistically significant. For the Caribbean group, all three means of standardising for socio-economic position reduce the relative risk to a level that is barely significantly greater than that for the white group. For the Indian or African Asian group, standardising for occupational class and tenure again makes little difference, but controlling for standard of living brings the risk very nearly to statistically significantly lower than that of the white group.

**Table 6.14    Relative risk of reported fair, poor, or very poor health compared with whites, standardised by socio-economic factors**

|  | Indian or African Asian | Pakistani or Bangladeshi | Caribbeans |
|---|---|---|---|
| **Type of standardisation** |  |  |  |
| Age and gender | 0.99 (0.9-1.1) | 1.45 (1.3-1.6) | 1.25 (1.10-1.4) |
| Class, age and gender | 1.00 (0.9-1.1) | 1.36 (1.2-1.5) | 1.15 (1.03-1.3) |
| Tenure, age and gender | 1.04 (0.9-1.2) | 1.45 (1.3-1.6) | 1.17 (1.04-1.3) |
| Standard of living, age and gender | 0.94 (0.9-1.04) | 1.24 (1.1-1.4) | 1.15 (1.03-1.3) |

## Heart disease

Table 6.15 shows the relative risk compared with those in the white group of having a diagnosis of angina or heart disease. Given the findings from the immigrant mortality analyses (Marmot et al., 1984; Balarajan, 1991; Harding and Maxwell, 1997), the two South Asian groupings are of most interest here. As with the previous table, controlling for occupational class or tenure makes little difference to the data presented, although, if anything, such controls increase the relative risk of the South Asian groups. However, controlling for standard of living makes an important difference. The Indian or African Asian group now has a significantly lower risk than the white group, while the risk for the Pakistani or Bangladeshi group is also lowered and is now no longer significantly greater than the rate in the white group.

**Table 6.15    Relative risk of diagnosed angina or heart attack[1] compared with whites, standardised by socio-economic factors**

|  | Indian or African Asian | Pakistani or Bangladeshi | Caribbeans |
|---|---|---|---|
| **Type of standardisation** |  |  |  |
| Age and gender | 0.77 (0.5-1.1) | 1.50 (1.1-2.0) | 0.95 (0.6-1.4) |
| Class, age and gender | 0.92 (0.6-1.3) | 1.49 (1.1-2.1) | 1.05 (0.7-1.6) |
| Tenure, age and gender | 0.85 (0.6-1.2) | 1.57 (1.2-2.1) | 0.93 (0.6-1.4) |
| Standard of living, age and gender | 0.67 (0.5-0.96) | 1.24 (0.9-1.7) | 1.02 (0.7-1.5) |

1 In addition to 'heart attack', the question wording added 'including a heart murmur, a damaged heart or a rapid heart'.

Table 6.16 includes respondents who reported suffering from severe chest pain in addition to those who reported a diagnosis of heart disease. Once again, controlling for occupational class and tenure makes little difference to the relative risks of the two South Asian groups, while controlling for standard of living considerably reduces the risk for both of them. However, for this outcome the risk for Indian or African Asian people is just outside being significantly lower than that for white people, and the risk for Pakistani or Bangladeshi people is still just significantly greater.

**Table 6.16    Relative risk of diagnosed heart disease[1] or severe chest pain compared with whites, standardised by socio-economic factors[2]**

|                                 | Indian or African Asian | Pakistani or Bangladeshi | Caribbeans        |
| ------------------------------- | ----------------------- | ------------------------ | ----------------- |
| **Type of standardisation**     |                         |                          |                   |
| Age and gender                  | 0.95 (0.7-1.2)          | 1.88 (1.5-2.4)           | 0.96 (0.7-1.3)    |
| Class, age and gender           | 0.93 (0.7-1.2)          | 1.59 (1.2-2.0)           | 0.85 (0.6-1.2)    |
| Tenure, age and gender          | 1.05 (0.8-1.4)          | 1.87 (1.5-2.4)           | 0.92 (0.7-1.3)    |
| Standard of living, age and gender | 0.78 (0.6-1.01)      | 1.37 (1.1-1.7)           | 0.89 (0.7-1.2)    |

1 In addition to 'heart attack', the question wording added 'including a heart murmur, a damaged heart or a rapid heart'.
2 Only those aged 40 or older are included here.

## Hypertension

Table 6.17 shows the relative risk of having a diagnosis of hypertension compared with the white group for each ethnic minority group once the various forms of standardisation had been carried out.

Interestingly, the pattern for the Caribbean group follows that for the South Asian groupings in the previous two tables, with controlling for occupational class increasing risk, controlling for tenure making no difference in risk, and controlling for standard of living both reducing their risk and bringing it close to being not significantly different from that of the white group. Controlling for standard of living also slightly reduces the risk for the Indian or African Asian and the Pakistani or Bangladeshi groups.

**Table 6.17    Relative risk of diagnosed hypertension compared with whites, standardised by socio-economic factors**

|                                 | Indian or African Asian | Pakistani or Bangladeshi | Caribbeans        |
| ------------------------------- | ----------------------- | ------------------------ | ----------------- |
| **Type of standardisation**     |                         |                          |                   |
| Age and gender                  | 0.64 (0.5-0.8)          | 0.94 (0.8-1.1)           | 1.49 (1.2-1.8)    |
| Class, age and gender           | 0.70 (0.6-0.9)          | 0.88 (0.7-1.1)           | 1.56 (1.3-1.9)    |
| Tenure, age and gender          | 0.68 (0.6-0.8)          | 0.95 (0.8-1.1)           | 1.42 (1.2-1.7)    |
| Standard of living, age and gender | 0.60 (0.5-0.7)       | 0.86 (0.7-1.04)          | 1.33 (1.1-1.6)    |

# Diabetes

Table 6.18, which focuses on diabetes, shows a similar pattern to previous tables. For all three ethnic minority groups, controlling for occupational class and tenure makes little difference, although for the Caribbean group applying the tenure controls leads to some reduction in risk. But for all of the ethnic minority groups, controlling for standard of living slightly reduces the risk of diabetes compared with the white group, although differences for this outcome still remain both statistically significant and large.

**Table 6.18   Relative risk of diabetes compared with whites, standardised by socio-economic factors**

|  | Indian or African Asian | Pakistani or Bangladeshi | Caribbeans |
|---|---|---|---|
| **Type of standardisation** | | | |
| Age and gender | 2.6 (1.7-3.9) | 4.9 (3.3-7.2) | 2.6 (1.6-4.0) |
| Class, age and gender | 3.1 (2.0-4.6) | 5.2 (3.4-7.8) | 2.8 (1.8-4.3) |
| Tenure, age and gender | 2.7 (1.8-4.1) | 4.8 (3.3-6.9) | 2.3 (1.4-3.6) |
| Standard of living, age and gender | 2.4 (1.6-3.6) | 4.1 (2.9-6.0) | 2.2 (1.4-3.4) |

# Respiratory disease

Table 6.19 includes respondents who reported that they had either a wheeze or had coughed up phlegm for at least three months of the year. These questions were only asked of half of the ethnic minority respondents, hence the relatively wide confidence limits shown in the table. The table shows that the effect of controlling for socio-economic group is small for all of the indicators of socio-economic position used and for all of the ethnic minority groups. However, the risk for all of the groups is smallest when standard of living is controlled for. For the Caribbean group, the relative risk compared with the white group of reporting respiratory symptoms is not statistically significant if the data are standardised according to occupational class and tenure, but if standard of living is controlled for, the relative risk for Caribbean people becomes, like that for those in the other ethnic minority groups, significantly lower.

**Table 6.19   Relative risk of wheezing or coughing up phlegm compared with whites, standardised by socio-economic factors**

|  | Indian or African Asian | Pakistani or Bangladeshi | Caribbeans |
|---|---|---|---|
| **Type of standardisation** | | | |
| Age and gender | 0.53 (0.4-0.6) | 0.65 (0.6-0.8) | 0.89 (0.7-1.05) |
| Class, age and gender | 0.53 (0.4-0.6) | 0.55 (0.5-0.7) | 0.86 (0.7-1.01) |
| Tenure, age and gender | 0.58 (0.5-0.7) | 0.65 (0.6-0.8) | 0.85 (0.7-1.01) |
| Standard of living, age and gender | 0.50 (0.4-0.6) | 0.50 (0.4-0.6) | 0.83 (0.7-0.98) |

# Neurotic depression

The effect of standardising for socio-economic position on differences in the estimated weekly prevalence of depression is shown in Table 6.20. For the Indian or African Asian group, controlling for occupational class and, particularly, for tenure led to an increase in relative risk compared with the white group, while controlling for standard of living led to a reduction in relative risk. For the Pakistani or Bangladeshi group, the table shows that controlling for socio-economic position made little difference, although reductions were present and greatest once standard of living had been controlled for. For the Caribbean group, controlling for both tenure and standard of living led to a reduction in relative risk compared with the white group, while controlling for occupational class made little difference.

**Table 6.20    Relative risk of depressive neurosis during the past week compared with whites, standardised by socio-economic factors**

| | Indian or African Asian | Pakistani or Bangladeshi | Caribbeans |
|---|---|---|---|
| **Type of standardisation** | | | |
| Age and gender | 0.71 (0.5-1.1) | 0.76 (0.5-1.2) | 1.48 (1.01-2.2) |
| Class, age and gender | 0.78 (0.5-1.2) | 0.69 (0.4-1.1) | 1.42 (0.96-2.1) |
| Tenure, age and gender | 0.93 (0.6-1.4) | 0.73 (0.5-1.1) | 1.28 (0.9-1.9) |
| Standard of living, age and gender | 0.62 (0.4-0.9) | 0.67 (0.4-1.02) | 1.33 (0.9-1.9) |

# Non-affective psychosis

Table 6.21 shows the estimated annual prevalence of non-affective psychosis. The findings are very similar to those for depression. Controlling for standard of living led to a reduction in relative risk for the Indian or African Asian group compared with the white group, but other socio-economic controls either resulted in no change (occupational class) or to an increase in relative risk (tenure). For the Pakistani or Bangladeshi group, controlling for occupational class and tenure led to small reductions in relative risk, while controlling for standard of living led to a larger reduction. And for the Caribbean group, controlling for all three socio-economic measures led to some reduction in relative risk. Here it is also interesting to note that Table 6.10 suggests that most of the difference between the Caribbean and white groups can be accounted for by the relatively high rate among non-manual Caribbean people. Rates for Caribbean people from households with no full-time worker and those that were manual were only slightly higher than those for equivalent white respondents, while the difference for those from non-manual households was fourfold.

**Table 6.21    Relative risk of non-affective psychosis during the past year compared with whites, standardised by socio-economic factors**

| | Indian or African Asian | Pakistani or Bangladeshi | Caribbeans |
|---|---|---|---|
| **Type of standardisation** | | | |
| Age and gender | 0.73 (0.4-1.5) | 0.67 (0.3-1.5) | 1.66 (0.8-3.3) |
| Class, age and gender | 0.71 (0.4-1.4) | 0.58 (0.3-1.3) | 1.55 (0.8-3.0) |
| Tenure, age and gender | 0.90 (0.5-1.8) | 0.63 (0.3-1.4) | 1.58 (0.8-3.1) |
| Standard of living, age and gender | 0.66 (0.3-1.4) | 0.53 (0.2-1.2) | 1.56 (0.8-3.0) |

## Summary

The data presented in Tables 6.14 to 6.21 clearly show that if we wish to examine whether differences in socio-economic position make an important contribution to ethnic differences in health, we must be careful about the indicators of socio-economic position we use. Although the index of standard of living is far from perfect in this respect – see Table 6.13, which shows socio-economic variations within bands of standard of living, and note that it does not include a lifetime estimate of socio-economic position, which may be of great importance for particular outcomes such as diabetes (Davey Smith et al., 1997) – it is an improvement on the traditional indicators of socio-economic position, occupational class and tenure, that have been used both for the general population and for comparisons across ethnic groups. The difficulties with the use of these traditional indicators for making comparisons across ethnic group comparisons are clearly illustrated in Table 6.12.

The data in Table 6.1, taken together with those shown in Table 6.12, suggest that all of the ethnic minority groups considered in this chapter (Caribbean, Indian or African Asian, and Pakistani or Bangladeshi) are relatively disadvantaged compared with the white group, although the degree of disadvantage varies across these groups. Consequently, if socio-economic position does contribute to the ethnic differences in health reported here, controlling for socio-economic position should reduce the relative risk of ill-health for all of these ethnic minority groups compared with whites. If the age- and gender-standardised data are compared with the data that also include controls for standard of living in Tables 6.14 to 6.21, i.e. if the top and bottom rows of these tables are compared, this is the pattern that is consistently repeated. For only one outcome and one ethnic minority group, the relative risk for Caribbean compared with white people to report a diagnosis of heart disease, is the risk once standard of living is controlled greater than that when only age and gender are considered. In every other case the risk is reduced, although in some instances the reduction is small.

In addition, despite the limitations of the standard of living index, in all cases, except diabetes, relative risks that were statistically significantly greater compared with whites are either no longer or only just significantly different once standard of living is controlled for. This does suggest that socio-economic position makes an important contribution to ethnic inequalities in health. Importantly, this applies to the greater risk of heart disease that those in the Pakistani or Bangladeshi group reported and the greater risk of hypertension that was found in the Caribbean group, both of which others have argued are genetic effects (e.g. Wild and McKeigue, 1997). It is also worth pointing out that some differences that were not statistically significantly different from the white population when only gender and age are considered do become significantly lower when standard of living is also considered. An important example of this is the risk of diagnosed heart disease for the Indian or African Asian group and respiratory symptoms for the Caribbean group.

## CONCLUSION

The data presented in this chapter show that, as for the general population, socio-economic position is an important predictor of health for ethnic minority groups. Tables 6.2 to 6.8 showed that for both general health indicators and those that reflected particular physical conditions, people in poorer socio-economic groups had poorer health in each ethnic group. A similar pattern was found for the mental health outcomes, shown in Tables 6.9 and 6.10, for the white, Caribbean and Indian or African Asian groups. Although there was no socio-economic gradient for either mental health outcome for the Pakistani or Bangladeshi group, evidence on differences between those who were migrants and non-migrants in Chapter 5 raises the possibility that this may have been a consequence of methodological difficulties. This issue has been investigated in these data elsewhere, and multivariate models showed clear socio-economic gradients in mental health outcomes for those in the South Asian group when a migration variable was included (Nazroo, 1997b).

In contrast to the clear socio-economic gradients in health outcomes shown here, as described earlier, Marmot et al.'s (1984) classic study of immigrant mortality came to the conclusion that social class gradients in mortality rates did not exist for migrants from either the Caribbean or the Indian sub-continent. As suggested earlier, the discrepancy between the conclusions reached here and those reached by Marmot et al. (1984) need careful consideration. Here it is worth highlighting differences between the approaches of the two studies that lead to their data not being directly comparable:

- The definition of ethnicity used here is based on country of family origin, while that in Marmot et al.'s (1984) study is based on country of birth.
- Data used here are based on self-reports of morbidity, or diagnosis of morbidity, while Marmot et al., (1984) used mortality. While the two are related, there are also potential important differences, as discussed in Chapter 2.

- Socio-economic position was defined here using *current* occupation, tenure, or standard of living, while Marmot et al. (1984) used occupation as recorded at time of death. The use of occupation as recorded on death certificates may cause particular problems for immigrant mortality data due to the inflating of occupational status. (According to Townsend and Davidson (1982), occupation is recorded as the 'skilled' job held for most of the individual's life rather than the 'unskilled' job held in the last few years of life.) This will be a particularly significant problem for such data if migration to Britain was associated with significant downward social mobility for members of ethnic minority groups, a process that both Smith (1977) and Heath and Ridge (1983) have documented. The occupation recorded on the death certificates of migrants, consequently, may well be an inaccurate reflection of experience in Britain prior to death. In addition, given the socio-economic profile of ethnic minority groups in Britain, this inflation of occupational status would only need to happen in relatively few cases for the figures representing the small population in higher classes to be distorted. For example, Table 3.7 in Marmot et al. (1984) shows that in 1970–72 in the class I group only 212 deaths occurred among those born in the Indian sub-continent and only 37 occurred among those born in the Caribbean.
- Finally, differences between the data reported here and by Marmot et al. (1984) may reflect genuine differences between the populations studied. Important cohort effects may have operated between the exclusively immigrant ethnic minority population who had their health assigned by mortality rates, and the ethnic minority population interviewed about 20 years later that included both migrants and those born in Britain, and who had their health assessed by self-reported morbidity.

These points not only suggest that the data used in the two studies are not necessarily directly comparable, they also suggest that the data used here are in a number of ways an improvement on the mortality data used by Marmot et al. (1984), being nationally representative of the ethnic minority groups used, having more accurate assessments of socio-economic position and ethnicity, and, consequently, being less likely to suffer from artefact effects.

The data presented here also showed that traditional indicators of socio-economic position, such as occupational class and tenure, are inappropriate for adjusting for socio-economic effects when making comparisons across ethnic groups. Table 6.11 shows that within particular socio-economic bands members of ethnic minority groups were worse off than white people; for example, within particular occupational class bands those in the Pakistani or Bangladeshi group had half the income of those in the white group. This lends support to Kaufman et al.'s (1997, 1998) criticisms of attempts to control for socio-economic effects to simulate randomisation when making comparisons across ethnic groups. So, not surprisingly, Tables 6.14 to 6.21 show that for a variety of general and specific indicators of health, controlling for occupational class or tenure made little or no difference to ethnic inequalities in health. However, controlling for an indicator of socio-economic position that is more sensitive to ethnic differences, standard of living, led to a reduction in the relative risk to be in the illness category for ethnic minority people compared with white people in all but one outcome for only one of the ethnic minority groups.

Again, it is worth pointing out that 'controlling' for socio-economic position cannot be completely done, even if specifically tailored indicators such as standard of living are used. Table 6.13 shows that within bands of standard of living important differences in income between ethnic groups remained. In addition to this, it is also important to recall that taking account of socio-economic position only deals with part of the structural disadvantage faced by ethnic minority groups. Other important features of the lives of ethnic minority groups may adversely effect their health in comparison to the white population, such as their experiences of racism and discrimination (Karlsen and Nazroo, 2001), their perception of the inequality they face in their lives, and their geographical concentration in urban locations. It is likely that differences in the social experiences between ethnic minority and majority groups cannot be reduced to indicators of socio-economic position based on occupation, deprivation or consumption. All of this reinforces Kaufman et al.'s (1998) comments on the multi-dimensional nature of the disadvantage faced by ethnic minority people and the great difficulty in making sufficient adjustments across all of these dimensions in order to simulate randomisation. Despite this, not only were differences between the white and ethnic minority samples reduced once standard of living had been taken into account; in many instances important differences, such as those for diagnosed heart disease, became no longer statistically significant.

The conclusions to be reached, consequently, are that socio-economic position is an important predictor of health within all ethnic groups and it also makes an important contribution to the pattern of ethnic inequalities in health that have been reported both here and elsewhere.

# Chapter Seven

# Conclusion

In the introduction to this volume, the context of this survey was fully described. Some of the issues raised there are worth reiterating, prior to an overview of key findings, following which approaches to understanding ethnic inequalities in health will be reconsidered.

When placing this work in the context of the wider literature, it should be recognised that this survey is unique in terms of its coverage of ethnic minority populations, the health assessments included in the study, and its coverage of other features of the lives of ethnic minority people in Britain. Most general population surveys do not contain sufficient numbers of ethnic minority people for their samples to be representative of ethnic minority groups, or for the relevant issues to be fully investigated. Health surveys that specifically explore issues to do with ethnicity are either regional (e.g. Pilgrim et al., 1993; Williams et al., 1993), or, if national, typically only sample from areas where relatively large numbers of ethnic minority people live (typically 10 per cent or more, e.g. Rudat, 1994; Johnson et al., 2000). The only other study that has a truly nationally representative sample of ethnic minority people, the 1999 Health Survey for England (Erens et al., 2001), has very limited coverage of issues relevant to understanding the reasons for ethnic inequalities in health (although it has good coverage of disease, and, uniquely, includes ethnic minority children (Nazroo et al., 2001)). The most influential work in the epidemiological investigation of ethnic difference in health has, of necessity, relied on immigrant mortality data (Marmot et al., 1984; Balarajan and Bulusu, 1990; Balarajan, 1996; Harding and Maxwell, 1997; Maxwell and Harding, 1998). However, these have several important drawbacks described earlier: they use a one-dimensional indicator of health; they have a limited and crude coverage of ethnic minority populations; and they have an inadequate coverage of possible explanatory factors for the observed relationships. All of these limitations should lead to the conclusions drawn from such data being treated with a significant amount of caution.

There are important additional methodological problems with studies on ethnic differences in mental health. Almost all of them have been based on treatment statistics, and often they are based only on data on hospital admissions. Such data contain a number of difficulties that limit our ability to generalise from them (and which were discussed in detail in the introduction). Most important here is that differences in the pathways into care for different ethnic groups, rather than differences in rates of illness, may have influenced the pattern of findings reported. For example, African Caribbean people with a psychosis may be more likely than equivalent white people to end up in hospital and, in contrast, South Asian people with a common mental disorder (such as depression) may be less likely to do so. One possible reason for differences in pathways into care is that they are a consequence of cultural differences in the expression and experience of mental illness leading to under-treatment among some ethnic groups, a concern that applies particularly to South Asian people and depression (Kleinman, 1987). Alternatively, it is possible that patterns of racialisation could lead to the over-diagnosis and overestimation of mental illness in some groups, particularly as far as African Caribbean people and psychosis are concerned (Sashidaran, 1993). For example, there is growing evidence suggesting that African Caribbean patients are more likely than white patients to be treated coercively for psychotic illnesses and that this might not be appropriate (Harrison et al., 1989; McKenzie et al., 1995; Davies et al., 1996). Regardless of these possibilities, the quality and interpretation of data based on treatment statistics alone is always open to question, because of class, gender and regional differences, in addition to ethnic differences, in patterns and opportunities for consultation (Blane et al., 1996; McKinlay, 1996).

Given these limitations with other data sources, the Fourth National Survey can be considered an important benchmark in work on ethnic inequalities in health. This study comprised a large nationally representative survey of the main ethnic minority groups in Britain, together with a comparison survey of the white population. The survey was community-based, so not dependent on the prior identification of potentially ill people. It also contained a large enough sample in the white, Caribbean and South Asian groups to allow the pattern of findings based on treatment and mortality statistics to be tested. And it covered a range of other topics concerning the lives and experiences of the respondents, which consequently meant that it offered an opportunity to explore the important question of whether the various forms of social disadvantage faced by ethnic minority people contributed to their risk of illness.

However, two notes of caution need to be sounded in the interpretation of the results presented, both of which are a result of the reliance on a standardised cross-sectional survey instrument. First, the assessments of health are based entirely on self-reports. None of these measures has been clinically validated for cross-cultural research. Indeed such self-reports could be related to cultural and language differences. Consequently, their accuracy could be biased by the ethnicity of the respondent, which could then lead to an inaccurate representation of ethnic difference in health. Although we should take seriously the possibility that the data presented are the result of an artefact in reporting style or opportunity for diagnosis, some reassurance about the validity of the measures of physical health used can be drawn from the fact that within ethnic groups the expected distribution of health across factors such as age, gender and class was found, and that across ethnic groups different types of health assessment (for example, questions on diagnosis and questions on symptoms) and the assessment of different but related dimensions of health (for example, smoking and respiratory symptoms) showed consistent patterns.

In this regard a particular set of problems existed for the Fourth National Survey's assessment of *mental* illness. At the main interview stage the assessment was limited both by time constraints and by the skills of lay interviewers, who were trained in social rather than psychiatric research. To address this problem, the mental health assessment in the Fourth National Survey followed a similar design to that used in the National Psychiatric Morbidity Survey (Meltzer et al., 1995): respondents who appeared to be possibly suffering from a depressive or psychotic disorder on the basis of their responses to structured questions were recontacted and underwent a clinical interview based on the PSE. This enabled the relationship between responses to the questions in the initial interview to be compared with the PSE-derived diagnostic class that applied to the respondents who were followed up. The results of this comparison then allowed an examination of the cross-cultural validity of these assessments of mental disorder and for the CIS-R and PSQ responses to be used to estimate the prevalence of neurotic depression and non-affective psychosis in each group.

The second note of caution concerns the interpretation of the suggested explanatory relationships. The cross-sectional nature of the survey means that causal direction can only be assumed from these data. So, although they do show clear relationships between suggested explanatory factors and ethnic inequalities in health, the direction of the relationships shown cannot be determined. Some confidence can be drawn from the fact that studies in other populations have repeatedly shown similar relationships (Townsend and Davidson, 1982; Blaxter 1987; Townsend et al., 1988; Blaxter, 1990; Davey Smith et al., 1990b; Haynes, 1991) and the causal directions assumed in this report have been generally acknowledged as, and shown to be, appropriate (Davey Smith et al., 1990a; Kuh and Wadsworth, 1993; Bartley, 1994; Benzeval et al., 1995; Department of Health, 1995).

## KEY FINDINGS

The following provides an overview of the findings shown in earlier chapters of this volume, structured by illness 'type'. The first section provides a summary of the findings on general health and how this is patterned across ethnic groups, so provides an overview of health disadvantage and how this may be related to the position of ethnic minority groups in Britain.

# General health

Chapter 3 showed the large burden of ill-health faced by members of some ethnic minority groups, despite their relatively young age profile compared with whites. More than a third of people in the Pakistani or Bangladeshi and Caribbean groups reported that they had fair, poor, or very poor health and 20 per cent of people in the Pakistani or Bangladeshi group said that their performance of moderately exerting activities, such as climbing one flight of stairs, was in some way limited by their health. In contrast, only just over a quarter of Indian or African Asian people reported that they had either fair, poor, or very poor health. Age-standardised relative risks confirmed there were important differences in the experiences of ethnic minority groups. For example, while the Pakistani or Bangladeshi and Caribbean groups were statistically significantly more likely than whites to report fair, poor, or very poor health (50 per cent more likely for the former and 30 per cent more likely for the latter), the Indian or African Asian group had a very similar rate to whites. The pattern of findings was consistent across all but one of the assessments of general health used[1] and very similar to those from the only comparable data sources, the 1991 Census (Nazroo, 1997a) and the 1999 Health Survey for England (Erens et al., 2001).

Chapters 4 and 5 explored the relationship between self-assessed general health and ethnic group further. Chapter 5 showed that the differences between ethnic minority groups and whites could not be attributed to disadvantage experienced in the country of birth – those that were born in Britain or migrated at an early age were, if anything, more likely than those who migrated aged 11 or older to report that their health was fair, poor, or very poor. In addition, Chapter 4 showed that if ethnic sub-groups were considered, important differences within particular ethnic minority groups emerged, reinforcing the suggestion of a lack of uniformity of risk within particular ethnic groups. Chapter 6 used indicators of socio-economic position to explore further the variation in risk within ethnic groups. For each of the ethnic groups considered, there was a strong and statistically significant relationship between socio-economic position and reported fair, poor, or very poor health. Moreover, once the difficulties with controlling for socio-economic position across ethnic groups had been partially addressed, the relative risk for members of all of the ethnic minority groups compared with whites to report fair, poor, or very poor health was reduced, although differences between the Pakistani or Bangladeshi and white groups, and the Caribbean and white groups, remained statistically significant.

The data on general health from this survey clearly show that levels of ill-health vary markedly across ethnic minority groups, as well as between ethnic

---

1   The only exception to this was the question on long-standing illness, which others (Pilgrim et al., 1993; Rudat, 1994) and the data shown in Chapter 3 suggest is not a valid indicator for exploring ethnic difference in health. Interestingly, an extension of the question so that it only included long-standing illnesses *that limited work* did, in contrast, show the general pattern just reported.

minority and majority groups. The implication is that studies that have generalised from ethnic sub-groups to a wider group, such as from Bangladeshis to South Asians (McKeigue et al., 1988), will be misleading, as will those that use crude ethnic groupings that are very heterogeneous, such as all ethnic minorities (Benzeval et al., 1992; Gould and Jones, 1996), or all South Asians (Marmot et al., 1984; Balarajan and Bulusu, 1990). The data presented in this volume also strongly indicate that a key factor in explaining these ethnic inequalities in general health are the differing overall socio-economic positions of different ethnic groups. Both within and across ethnic groups, socio-economic position showed a strong relationship with health status.

## Cardiovascular disease

The data on coronary heart disease presented in this volume also showed important differences between ethnic minority groups and contradicted many of the assumptions that have underpinned previous work in this area. Most work on ethnic difference in heart disease has considered South Asians to be a group that is uniformly at greater risk of coronary heart disease (e.g. McKeigue et al., 1989; McKeigue, 1992 and 1993; McKeigue and Sevak, 1994; Gupta et al., 1995). However, the data presented here showed important differences in the rates both of diagnosis and of symptoms of coronary heart disease across the groups that comprise South Asians. For example, among those aged 40 or more, almost 25 per cent of Pakistani or Bangladeshi people reported that they had either severe chest pain or diagnosed heart disease, compared with 12 per cent of Indian or African Asian people. In the comparison with the white population, while the South Asian group as a whole had a higher risk of having either a diagnosis or symptoms suggestive of heart disease, this greater risk only applied to the Pakistani or Bangladeshi group, with the Indian or African Asian group having the same risk as whites – findings that are consistent with those on self-reported diagnoses of Ischaemic Heart Disease and ECG changes in the 1999 Health Survey for England (Erens et al., 2001). Additionally, an examination of religious sub-groups within the Indian or African Asian category suggested that rates of heart disease were 22 times higher among Muslims than among Hindus.

Although these findings do contradict the assumptions underlying much of the work in this area, they were consistent across age and gender groups and across types of question used.[2] In fact, a careful inspection of earlier work that has attempted to explore differences between South Asian groups in this

---

2   Questions were asked on diagnosis of angina, diagnosis of heart disease, experience of chest pain and severity of chest pain. The question on diagnosis of heart disease included 'a heart murmur, a damaged heart or a rapid heart', which would cover conditions beyond coronary heart disease. However, the consistency of response across the questions on diagnosis and those on symptoms suggests that the inclusion of the additional items was not too misleading.

respect, despite the difficulties of the task given the quality of data available, also suggests that there may be important differences between South Asian groups for coronary heart disease. Table III of Balarajan et al. (1984) suggests that Muslims had a greater proportional mortality ratio for death from myocardial infarction than any other South Asian group (although this paper is often cited as demonstrating uniform risk across South Asian groups, e.g. McKeigue et al., 1989 and 1991, and Gupta et al., 1995, all of which cite this study as showing no differences, presumably because of assumptions that earlier studies that had combined South Asian groups had not been misleading). And, while the analysis of the most recent immigrant mortality data still showed a relatively high standardised mortality rate from coronary heart disease for those born in the Indian sub-continent overall (over the period 1988–92 and for those aged 20–69 it was 138 for men and 143 for women), this risk varied greatly across the country of birth groups, and in a way that was not consistent between men and women (Balarajan, 1996). Both men and women born in Sri Lanka and East Africa had a similar risk to those born in England and Wales, while men born in India had a lower standardised mortality rate (137) than those born in Pakistan (142), who in turn had a lower standardised mortality rate than those born in Bangladesh (147), and, in contrast, women born in India had a higher standardised mortality rate (158) than those born in Pakistan or Bangladesh, for whom the standardised mortality rate was similar to or lower than that for women born in England and Wales (104 and 80 respectively). This pattern is partly consistent with the findings reported here, but does contain some differences. Inconsistencies between immigrant mortality data and the morbidity data used here need to be interpreted in the light of differences between mortality and morbidity health assessments, which were outlined in Chapter 2. In particular, it is worth considering evidence that suggests that survival rates following myocardial infarction are higher for better-off socio-economic groups (Morrison et al., 1997) and for whites compared with South Asian people (Wilkinson et al., 1996; Shaukat et al., 1997).

Clearly such findings suggest that explanations for ethnic differences in coronary heart disease that are founded on the belief that South Asians have a shared greater risk, such as the insulin resistance syndrome hypothesis, should be rejected.[3] (Although, of course, this does not mean that insulin resistance does not have a potential role in the aetiology of coronary heart disease, simply that it cannot explain the uncovered ethnic difference.) Somewhat surprisingly, given the conclusions reached by others working in

---

3   However, it is worth considering the ability of the insulin resistance hypothesis to survive evidence that showed that Caribbean people had high rates of non-insulin dependent diabetes and low rates of coronary heart disease. Its proponents (e.g. Shaukat and Cruickshank, 1993) did this by suggesting that the high rates of diabetes might be a result of insulin deficiency rather than insulin resistance for Caribbean people, or that the component of insulin that caused coronary heart disease for South Asian people was not to be found in 'Caribbean' insulin.

this field (McKeigue et al., 1989), when the relationship between socio-economic position and coronary heart disease was explored, it was found that within ethnic groups there was a strong relationship between them that was in many instances statistically significant. Some support for this finding can be drawn from two studies. The first, in a rural location in western India, also showed a strong relationship between socio-economic position and coronary heart disease (Gupta et al., 1994). The second reported that the risk of coronary heart disease in South India was related to low birthweight and low maternal body weight, leading the authors to conclude that poor maternal nutrition may have been significant (Stein et al., 1996). In addition, once socio-economic position had been partially controlled for in this study, the risk of both diagnosed heart disease and symptoms suggestive of heart disease compared with whites dropped for all ethnic minority groups, and the former was no longer statistically significant for the Pakistani or Bangladeshi group. Again, the suggestion is that much of the ethnic variation in heart disease reported here could be attributed to differences in the socio-economic position between different ethnic minority groups.

The data on the reporting of a diagnosis of hypertension on the whole followed the pattern shown in previous studies (Marmot et al., 1984; Balarajan, 1991), with Caribbean people reporting higher rates of diagnosed hypertension than any other ethnic group. However, in contrast to the immigrant mortality data, the greater risk in comparison with white people applied only to women in the Caribbean group and did not apply to any of the South Asian groups. In fact, Indian or African Asian people appeared to have a lower risk than whites. Given that the questions used relied solely on the respondent having had hypertension diagnosed, and that hypertension is an asymptomatic condition so could only be identified if a screening opportunity arose, the accuracy of the data presented is questionable. However, they are consistent with those on measured hypertension from the 1999 Health Survey for England (Erens et al., 2001). Chapter 6 showed once again that within each ethnic group there was an inverse relationship between socio-economic position and the rate of diagnosis of hypertension, which in many cases was statistically significant. In addition, once socio-economic position had been partially controlled for, the relative risk of ethnic minority compared with white respondents to report a diagnosis of hypertension was reduced in every instance.

## Diabetes

For diabetes, ethnic differences in this study closely followed the pattern found in immigrant mortality data and other studies of diabetes in ethnic minority groups (Marmot et al., 1984; Balarajan and Bulusu, 1990; McKeigue et al., 1991; Erens et al., 2001). All of the ethnic minority groups had a much greater risk of a diagnosis of diabetes than whites. There were also important differences between ethnic minority groups, with men in the Pakistani or

Bangladeshi group having higher rates than men in the Indian or African Asian and Caribbean groups, and women in the Pakistani or Bangladeshi and Caribbean groups having higher rates than women in the Indian or African Asian group. In terms of an illness burden, diabetes is clearly a serious problem for ethnic minority groups. Despite the relatively young age profile of these groups, as many as one in thirteen of the Pakistani or Bangladeshi respondents, one in seventeen of the Caribbean respondents, and one in twenty of the Indian or African Asian respondents reported that they had a diagnosis of diabetes.

As for other health outcomes, within ethnic groups there was an inverse relationship between risk of having diagnosed diabetes and socio-economic position. However, uniquely among the outcomes considered here, once socio-economic position had been partially controlled for using the indicator of standard of living, the differences between the white group and all of the ethnic minority groups in the rate of diagnosis of diabetes remained large, although the risk of such a diagnosis was reduced.

## Respiratory symptoms

The coverage of symptoms suggestive of respiratory illness in this survey focused on questions asking about wheezing or coughing up phlegm. The responses to these questions illustrated that, unlike other health assessments used in this survey, ethnic minority respondents were less likely than whites to report these symptoms, with rates for both of the South Asian groups being significantly lower than those for whites, and those for Caribbean people being close to significantly lower. This is also consistent with immigrant mortality data, which show that those born in South Asia and the Caribbean have lower mortality rates from chronic respiratory conditions, a finding that the authors attributed to the low rates of smoking among ethnic minority groups (Marmot et al., 1984).

However, the data presented by Rudat (1994), in the 1999 Health Survey for England (Erens et al., 2001), and those reported here (described in more detail shortly) showed that significant numbers of people in some ethnic minority groups do smoke. Not surprisingly, for all ethnic groups smoking was highly related to the rate of reporting these respiratory symptoms, with white smokers being 50 per cent and ethnic minority smokers being on average 80 per cent more likely than their non-smoking counterparts to report these symptoms. In support of the hypothesis that differences in the risk of reporting respiratory symptoms across ethnic groups were the result of differences in rates of smoking, the age-standardised relative risks showed that ethnic minority respondents who smoked had roughly the same risk as their white equivalents. However, non-smokers in the two South Asian groups still had a lower rate of reporting respiratory symptoms than their white counterparts.

Once again, for all ethnic groups the rate of reporting these symptoms was strongly and significantly related to socio-economic position. Also, once socio-economic position had been partially controlled for, the risk for all ethnic minority groups compared with whites to have reported these symptoms became even smaller.

# Smoking

Smoking rates varied markedly by both ethnicity and gender. Women from the South Asian groups had very low rates of smoking, and only about one in six of Indian or African Asian men reported that they currently smoked. In contrast, almost a third of men in the Pakistani or Bangladeshi group reported that they currently smoked (if this group is separated, 44 per cent of Bangladeshi men reported being current smokers (see Nazroo, 1997a)). Smoking rates were also high among Caribbean people, but did not show a large gender difference: a third of Caribbean men and a quarter of Caribbean women reported that they currently smoked. Among the white respondents there was no gender difference in rates of smoking, with around a quarter of both men and women reporting that they currently smoked. These findings are similar (although the rates are not identical) to those reported by Rudat (1994) and in the 1999 Health Survey for England (Erens et al., 2001). Worryingly, while half of those white respondents who had ever smoked reported that they had given up, this was only the case for about one in five of smokers in the Indian or African Asian and Caribbean groups, and only one in eight Pakistani or Bangladeshi smokers had given up.

Smoking appeared to be related to age on migration to Britain. For all ethnic minority groups, those who were born in Britain or who had migrated at an early age were more likely than those who migrated aged 11 or older to have ever smoked. Many of these differences were statistically significant. Smoking was also inversely related to socio-economic position.

# Mental illness

*Estimated rates for the South Asian groups*

The apparent difference between the South Asian and white groups in the performance of the instruments used here to assess mental illness makes comparisons between these groups and assessments of actual rates of illness for South Asian people difficult to make. Evidence for the difference in their performance comes from a variety of findings in this study.

First, when making comparisons between the instruments used for the initial interview and the PSE used in the follow-up interview, the rate of confirmation of neurotic illness was much lower for the South Asian groups. It is possible that this reflected a genuine difference in rates of depression, but the fact that the confirmation rate for psychosis was identical for the white and South Asian groups, and that the lower confirmation rate for neurosis occurred in both the depression and the psychosis halves of the follow-up study, makes it possible that this was a consequence of a difference across ethnic groups in the performance of the mental health assessments used.

Second, the estimated prevalence of mental illness among the South Asian groups was much higher for those who were born in Britain or had migrated to Britain at an early age, compared with those who had migrated to Britain aged 11 or older. The estimated prevalence was also higher for South Asian people who were fluent in English. However, when age on migration and fluency in English were considered at the same time, the suggestion was that the former was most important. If age on migration and fluency in English are considered as surrogate indicators for acculturation, those who were the most acculturated (i.e. those who were both non-migrants and fluent in English) had the highest rates for both of the indicators of mental illness considered, and this pattern was confirmed for other indicators of mental illness used in this study (Nazroo, 1997b). This is the pattern of findings that we would expect to find if there was a problem with the cross-cultural use of these instruments.

Finally, a debriefing of interviewers used for the follow-up PSE-based interview also suggested that the instruments did not perform quite as well as they could have. Interviewers reported difficulties with the translations they were given, that they themselves had difficulty translating concepts appropriately into South Asian languages, and that interviews with those who were not fluent in English took much longer than those with respondents who were fluent. This bears some similarity to the findings reported by researchers who have explored the cross-cultural relevance of western psychiatry and found that the expression of mental illness in South Asian groups had important differences from the western pattern (Krause, 1989; Fenton and Sadiq-Sangster, 1996).

Overall, this provides support for Kleinman's (1987) critique of cross-cultural research and suggests that the instruments used failed to assess accurately the prevalence of mental illness among South Asian groups. If this were the case, our best estimates would come from the rates identified for the non-migrant groups, which appear to be similar to those for the white group for both depression and psychosis.

On the other hand, if we believe that this evidence about the relative performance of the screening and validation instruments is not convincing and accept that the differences between the white and South Asian groups estimated here are genuine, the overall pattern that emerges is one of a relatively healthy South Asian population. All of the South Asian groups had lower rates of depression and psychosis, although the differences were greater for migrants than for non-migrants and for women than for men.

As for the white group, the Indian or African Asian group showed a clear socio-economic gradient in risk of both indicators of mental illness, and the expected gender difference in risk of depression (with women having higher rates than men). However, the Pakistani or Bangladeshi group showed neither the gender difference nor the socio-economic gradient. In fact, given the generally poor economic position of the Pakistani or Bangladeshi group, the low overall rate of detected mental illness for them is surprising. One explanation might lie in the nature of the social support available to members of these groups. For example, it is possible that the location of South Asian people in particular geographical areas gives them greater access to support networks, which help them to cope with the various forms of social disadvantage that they face in those locations (Halpern, 1993; Smaje, 1995a; Halpern and Nazroo, 2000).

Nevertheless, despite the lack of a socio-economic gradient within the Pakistani or Bangladeshi group, making a partial adjustment for socio-economic effects led to a large reduction in relative risk of both depression and psychosis for them compared with the white group. For the Indian or African Asian group, this adjustment did lead to a reduction in the relative risk of psychosis compared with the white group, but the reduction in relative risk of depression was small.

## *Estimated rates for the Caribbean group*

Although the annual prevalence of non-affective psychosis estimated here was higher for the Caribbean group compared with the white group, the difference was not as great as the three to five times higher rate that treatment statistics have suggested. The overall rate was less than twice as high and this difference was not statistically significant. In addition, all of the difference was a result of the higher rate among Caribbean women compared with white women. Rates for Caribbean men were the same as those for white men. Other work has suggested that hospital admissions for first-onset schizophrenia are particularly high among Caribbean men born in Britain (Harrison et al., 1988) and among young Caribbean men (Cochrane and Bal, 1989). There was no evidence here to support either of these propositions. There was no difference between migrant and non-migrant members of the Caribbean group in the estimated annual prevalence of psychosis, this estimate did not vary greatly by age, and differences compared with the white group were at their smallest for the young. The lack of an age or cohort effect among this group also suggests that the greater risk that has been reported for them elsewhere was not a consequence of the exposure of a particular cohort to an environmental hazard, such as a prenatal infection (Glover, 1989).

Although these data do suggest that the rates of psychosis are not elevated in the Caribbean population to anything like the extent suggested by treatment statistics, there are a number of reasons why this interpretation might be mistaken. First, it is possible that the difference between the findings presented here and treatment statistics are a consequence of differences in the way in which the number of ill people is counted. Treatment statistics are based on *incidence* rates, counting each new case of psychosis within a specific time period. The rates presented here were based on the *prevalence* of cases of psychosis within a particular population and time period. Although this difference might at first sight seem trivial, if the time between onset and recovery from illness is different for compared populations, the different methods of counting would produce different findings. This is simply because the prevalence count would be relatively lower in the population that was recovering more quickly, as fewer of the onsets would still be ill in the time period that was covered. Consequently, if Caribbean people with psychosis were likely to have a shorter illness than their white counterparts, the prevalence rates presented here would have underestimated differences in incidence. There is some evidence to support this possibility: both McGovern et al. (1994) and McKenzie et al. (1995) showed that African Caribbean people with psychosis had a better prognosis than whites. But such differences would have to be fairly large to account for the relatively large differences in prevalence rates during a one-year period presented here and incidence rates presented elsewhere.

Second, it is possible that the community survey on which this study was based was more likely to have failed to include those who had a psychosis in the Caribbean group than in the white group. That is, the lower rate of psychosis among Caribbean people in this study might have been a consequence of an under-coverage of that group. The survey did not include institutions such as prisons and psychiatric hospitals, where young Caribbean men are more likely than any other group to be found, and such men may be more likely to suffer from a psychotic disorder (NACRO, 1995). And, as far as can be determined, refusal to participate in the study was highest among young Caribbean men. However, to explain the findings presented here, such an effect would have to be specific to young Caribbean men with a psychotic disorder and not be present for others with a psychotic disorder. No assessment was made at the point of attempted recruitment into the study, so it is impossible to determine whether this was the case, but because young men in the other ethnic minority groups also had higher refusal rates, the refusal rate for young Caribbean men was not surprisingly high.

Overall, then, it seems that while we should take these problems seriously, they were unlikely to have led to an underestimate in the rates of psychosis *specifically* for the Caribbean group. The parallel between the findings presented here and those for the Epidemiological Catchment Area (ECA) survey in the United States also lends support to the conclusions reached. Although treatment rates for psychosis among Black Americans are much higher than those for their white counterparts, the ECA survey showed that once age, gender, socio-economic position and marital status had been taken into account there were no differences between Blacks and whites in the prevalence of psychosis (Adebimpe, 1994).

Findings for the estimated weekly prevalence of neurotic depression among the Caribbean group also contradicted findings based on treatment statistics, which suggest that depression is less common among African Caribbean people than white people. Here the Caribbean group had a 60 per cent higher rate of depression than the white group and this difference was statistically significant. While the difference was present for both men and women, it was greater for men, with Caribbean men having twice the rate of white men.

A socio-economic gradient was apparent in the Caribbean group for both of the mental health outcomes, and making a partial adjustment for socio-economic differences reduced the relative risks for the Caribbean group compared with the white group. However, the socio-economic effect within the Caribbean groups was not statistically significant for either outcome.

## ETHNICITY AND HEALTH, APPROACHES TO UNDERSTANDING

### Untheorised ethnicity – epidemiological approaches

Researchers and commentators in the field of ethnicity and health seem divided over whether this work should be empirically or theoretically driven. Not surprisingly, those with a more epidemiological bent tend to argue for the former. If differences in rates of disease are present between groups that have been identified on the basis of an emergent 'ethnic' classification, these differences will provide a useful starting point for the identification and exploration of aetiological factors associated with those groups at higher risk. For example, Senior and Bhopal state:

> Epidemiology is the study of the distribution and determinants of disease. The main method of study, particularly for investigating the causes of disease, is to compare populations with different risks of disease. Ethnicity is a variable that is used increasingly to define populations for epidemiological studies (1994: 327).

A good example of this approach can be found in the work of McKeigue and colleagues (e.g. McKeigue et al., 1988, 1989 and 1991). This has a focus on a particular disease (CHD), rather than health *per se*, and uses the variation in the pattern of this disease across ethnic groups to provide clues for an understanding of its aetiology.

If the empirically driven approach of this work is accepted, criticism inevitably falls to the accuracy with which key 'ethnic' variables are measured. As I have described earlier, most epidemiological research on health and ethnicity has taken a crude approach to the allocation of individuals into ethnic groups, with much of the published data in this area allocating ethnicity according to country of birth, a strategy that is clearly limited. In addition, many studies use 'ethnic' groupings with quite inappropriate boundaries, such as Black or South Asian. The data are then interpreted as though the individuals within them are ethnically (i.e. genetically and culturally) homogeneous, even though such categories are heterogeneous, containing ethnic groups with different cultures, religions, migration histories, and geographical and socio-economic locations (see Bagley's, 1995, comments on a similar situation in the US).

Such criticisms lead to a focus on the technical problems with assigning individuals to ethnic categories during the research process, and a concern with such things as collecting sufficiently detailed information to differentiate between distinct groups; recording ethnic background in a consistent way; and dealing with issues such as mixed parentage (see Chaturvedi and McKeigue's, 1994, comments on the British data, and McKenney and Bennett's, 1994, comments on the data provided by the US Bureau of the Census). Solutions proposed involve more sensitive strategies for collecting information on ethnicity, for example by allowing individuals to define their ethnic group in their own terms. It is argued that this reduces the use of groups which are artefactual and without 'real' meaning (Aspinall, 1995) and avoids the construction of ethnic boundaries on the basis of the racist assumptions of researchers (Sheldon and Parker, 1992). (However, in most research using this model, including the 1991 and 2001 Census and one of the questions used in the study reported here, respondents are offered only a limited number of categories from which to choose.)

In apparent support of this position, the data presented here suggest that a more detailed approach to the assignment of individuals into ethnic groups reveals important additional differences between them. Figure 7.1 summarises some of the data presented earlier, using the ethnic categorisation based on the respondents' replies to the question on the country of their family origin. It shows the relative risk compared with whites for reporting fair, poor, or very poor general health for various ethnic minority groups. (In Figure 7.1, and some subsequent figures, the relative risk for each minority group is represented as the range within which there is a 95 per cent statistical probability of the true value lying, with the midpoint of the range also indicated. If the range does not cross the solid line at the value of '1', the value for the comparison white group, differences are, of course, statistically significant.) If the first three groups are examined, the figure shows that the use of an overall ethnic minority group obscures important differences between Caribbean and South Asian people. And, if the final three groups are compared, it shows that the use of an overall South Asian group obscures important differences between Indian or African Asian people on the one hand and Pakistani or Bangladeshi people on the other.

Figure 7.2 extends this exercise by summarising some of the data shown in Chapter 4. It shows how the rate of reported fair, poor, or very poor health compared with whites varied across four groups within the Indian or African Asian category, identified on the basis of religion, and suggests that the health experience of Indian and African Asian people varies along religious/cultural lines, with Muslims appearing to have worse health than the other groups (although the differences shown are not statistically significant).

Similar refinements can be made for the other ethnic groups included in Figure 7.1; for example the Caribbean group could be divided into African and Indian Caribbean groups, or by island of family origin, and the white group could be divided in many ways. The implication of these figures is that further

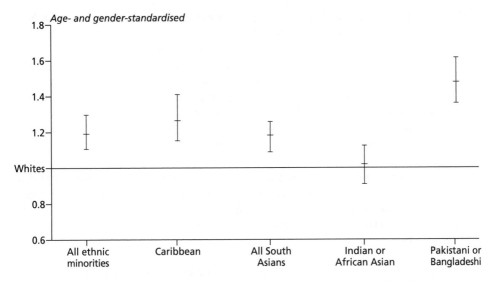

**Figure 7.1** Relative risk of reporting fair, poor or very poor health compared with whites

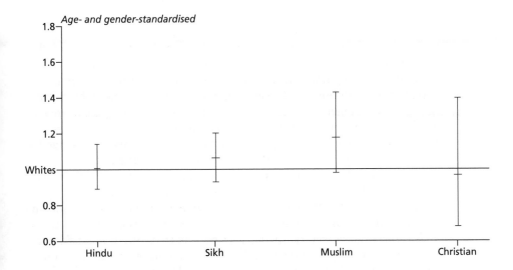

**Figure 7.2** Relative risk of reporting fair, poor or very poor health compared with whites – Indians only

refining the assessment of ethnicity used in epidemiological research will improve its power. More accurate assignments of ethnicity reveal additional differences and should allow a more careful generation of aetiological hypotheses and a more finely tuned programme for intervention.

It is here that the lack of theoretical work done by such researchers becomes important. Despite this lack, it is a mistake to assume that the process of identifying 'ethnic' groups is theoretically neutral (hence my use of the term 'untheorised' rather than atheoretical). Take the example of Marmot et al.'s (1984) immigrant mortality study, which in some ways could be seen as opportunistic, being based on the combination of country of birth data that was recorded at the 1971 Census and on death certificates. When discussing the rationale for their analysis, Marmot et al. have in mind a clear notion of the significance of their 'country of birth' variable:

> Comparisons of disease rates between immigrants and non-immigrants in the 'old' country, between immigrants and residents of the 'new' country, and between different immigrant groups in the new country have helped elucidate the relative importance of genetic and environmental factors in many diseases (1984: 4).

And, in his discussion of equivalent data relating to the period covered by the 1991 Census, Balarajan suggests that differences could be due to 'biological, cultural, religious, socio-economic or other environmental factors' (1996: 119).

However, in this work these explanatory factors are rarely assessed with any accuracy and the search for clues regarding aetiology is typically done with a focus on the assumed genetic or cultural characteristics of individuals within the ethnic group at greater risk. Consequently, explanations tend to fall to unmeasured genetic and cultural factors based on stereotypes, because such meanings are easily imposed on ethnic categorisations. Theory is brought in surreptitiously – ethnicity, however measured, equals genetic or cultural heritage and the inherent characteristics of the ethnic (minority) group are seen to be at fault and in need of rectifying (Sheldon and Parker, 1992). It is the ways in which ethnic and racial groups are constructed during this process, and the kinds of attributes focused on, that raise a concern with racialisation.

An example of this can be found in the well-publicised greater risk of 'South Asians' for CHD. A *British Medical Journal* editorial (Gupta et al., 1995) used research findings to attribute this problem to a combination of genetic and cultural factors that are apparently associated with being 'South Asian'. Concerning genetic factors, the suggestion was that 'South Asians' have a shared evolutionary history that involved adaptation 'to survive under conditions of periodic famine and low energy intake'. Here it is postulated that the evolutionary development of a 'thrifty' gene in South Asian populations, to deal with inconsistent food supplies, has led to a greater likelihood for people in these ethnic groups to develop non-insulin dependent diabetes in the form of 'insulin resistance syndrome', which apparently underlies the greater risk of CHD sustained by 'South Asians'. At a biomedical level, insulin resistance leads to an elevated concentration of insulin in plasma, which is then thought, either directly or through its effects on plasma concentrations of high-density-lipoprotein cholesterol and triglycerides, to increase the risk of atherosclerosis and consequent CHD (McKeigue et al., 1989). From this perspective 'South Asians' can be viewed as a genetically distinct group with a unique evolutionary history – a 'race'. In terms of cultural factors, the use of ghee in cooking, a lack of physical exercise and a reluctance to use health services were all mentioned – even though ghee is not used by all of the ethnic groups that comprise 'South Asians', and evidence suggests that 'South Asians' do understand the importance of exercise (Beishon and Nazroo, 1997) and do use medical services (Rudat, 1994; Nazroo, 1997a). It is important to note how the policy recommendations flowing from such an approach underline the extent to which the issue has become racialised. The authors of the editorial recommend that 'community leaders' and 'survivors' of heart attacks should spread the message among their communities and that 'South Asians' should be encouraged to undertake healthier lifestyles (Gupta et al., 1995). The problem is, apparently, viewed as something inherent to being 'South Asian', nothing to do with the context of the lives of 'South Asians' and as only solvable if 'South Asians' are encouraged to modify their behaviours to address their genetic and cultural weaknesses.

Another recent example can be found in relation to the higher mortality rates from hypertensive disease found among those born in the Caribbean and West Africa. In the conclusion to a paper that described variations in mortality rates in Britain by country of birth, the authors briefly discussed possible reasons for these higher death rates, stating:

> As migrants from the Caribbean and from west Africa have not shared a common environment for the past 300 years, a genetic explanation for the susceptibility to hypertension of people of west African descent is likely. The high mortality from diseases related to hypertension in migrants from west Africa does not support the hypothesis that black people in the United States are more prone to hypertension as a result of selective survival of slaves able to retain salt (Wild and McKeigue 1997: 709).

This clearly shows the form of reasoning taken by the authors. First, they consider environmental and genetic explanations to be alternatives when, of course, they may well operate synergistically. Second, they arrive at a genetic explanation by excluding other explanations, i.e. any redundant difference between ethnic groups must be a consequence of genetics, even though there is no direct evidence for genetic effects and the assessment of other effects can never be sufficiently sensitive or comprehensive (Kaufman et al., 1997 and 1998). Third, they envisage environment as operating in the past (over a 300-year period), perhaps through natural selection (hence the reference to salt retention and slaves). That is, environment is only important because over generations it leads to the differential selection of healthy or unhealthy genes in groups with different geographical roots. The shared current environment of disadvantage faced by Caribbean and African people living in London and Black people living in the United States is ignored.

A third example is the discussion of the high rates of suicide among young women born in South Asia provided by Soni-Raleigh and Balarajan (1992a), which is discussed in full in Chapter 1.

Given this risk of racialisation, it is not helpful to refine an ethnic classification scheme in a way that allows further assumptions to be made about the importance of culture and genetics when neither is measured and environment continues to be ignored. For example, the analysis in Chapter 3 showed that, while a South Asian group had a greater risk of indicators of CHD, once the group was broken down into constituent parts this only applied to the Pakistani or Bangladeshi group – Indian or African Asian people had the same rate as white people. In addition, within the Indian or African Asian group, Muslims had a high rate of indicators of CHD, while Hindus and Sikhs had low rates. While this approach is useful in uncovering the extent to which convenient assumptions of similarity within obviously heterogeneous groups were false, it could be suggested that these findings mean we can use the term 'Muslim heart disease', or 'Pakistani and Bangladeshi heart disease', rather than 'South Asian heart disease', to describe the situation. And explanations can be sought in assumptions about Muslim, Pakistani and Bangladeshi cultural practices or their shared evolutionary history. This potential results from the use of untheorised and apparently emergent ethnic classifications that allow ethnicity to be treated as a natural and fixed division between social groups, and the description of ethnic difference in health to become their explanation (Sheldon and Parker, 1992). Explanations are, consequently, based on cultural stereotypes or suppositions about genetic differences, rather than attempting to assess directly the nature and importance of such factors, the contexts in which they operate and their association with health outcomes.

So, in addition to refining our measurement of ethnicity, in order to progress we need to examine the degree to which the indicator used (country of birth, country of family origin, self-assigned ethnic group, etc.) reflects an underlying construct (Williams et al., 1994; Bagley, 1995; McKenzie and Crowcroft, 1996) – are we measuring genetics, biology, culture, lifestyle, the consequences of racialisation, socio-economic position etc., and are the indicators used appropriate to whichever of these we are concerned with?

## Ethnicity as structure – socio-economic position

One of the most consistent findings presented here is the strong relationship between socio-economic position and health across outcomes and for each ethnic group; the data strongly suggest that class effects are similar for ethnic minority and white people. Findings for one health outcome are presented graphically in Figure 7.3, which shows the strong relationship between class and reporting fair, poor, or very poor health for different ethnic groups.

Others have presented similar findings, both in smaller scale regional studies (e.g. Fenton et al., 1995) and in the most recent analysis of immigrant

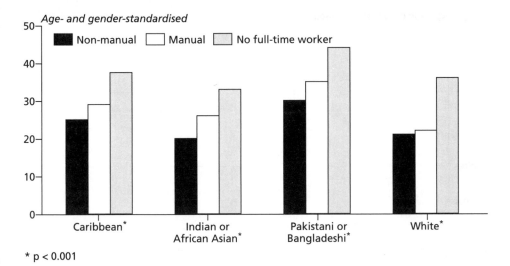

*Age- and gender-standardised*

Legend: Non-manual ■ | Manual □ | No full-time worker ▨

* p < 0.001

Figure 7.3    Reported fair, poor or very poor health by ethnic group and
class

mortality data (Harding and Maxwell, 1997). However, as described earlier, even after making adjustments for socio-economic position, such studies have continued to find differences in morbidity rates across ethnic groups and mortality rates across migrant groups. Indeed, a closer examination of Figure 7.3 supports this conclusion. For example, within each class group Pakistani or Bangladeshi people (suggested by Figure 7.1 to have the poorest health) were more likely than equivalent whites to report fair, poor, or very poor health, and the same is true for non-manual and manual Caribbean people (who overall also had poorer health than whites). The implication of both sets of data is that there remains some unidentified component of ethnicity that increases (some) ethnic minority groups' risk of poor health over and above socio-economic disadvantage. It is tempting to reduce this unexplained variance to assumed cultural or genetic factors.

However, this interpretation is misleading. Evidence presented earlier showed great variation in socio-economic position across ethnic groups within the *same* socio-economic bands. So ethnic minority people had a lower income than white people in the same class, unemployed ethnic minority people had been unemployed for longer than equivalent white people, and some ethnic minority groups had poorer quality housing than whites regardless of tenure (see Table 6.11). So, while standard indicators of socio-economic position may have some use for making comparisons *within* ethnic groups, they are of little use for 'controlling out' the impact of socio-economic differences when attempting to reveal a pure 'ethnic/race' effect.

Figure 7.4 provides additional support for this conclusion. It shows changes in the relative risk of reporting fair, poor, or very poor health for the

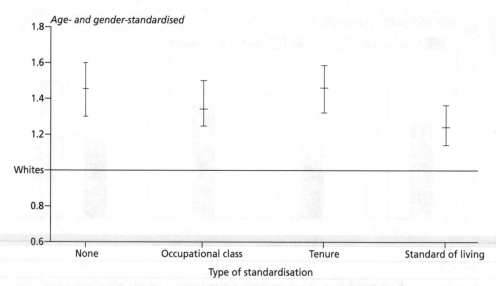

Figure 7.4    **Relative risk of fair, poor or very poor health standardised for socio-economic factors – Pakistani or Bangladeshi group compared with whites**

Pakistani or Bangladeshi group (the groups with the poorest health) compared with whites once the data had been standardised for a variety of socio-economic factors. Comparing the first bar with the second and third shows that standardising for class and tenure makes no difference. However, taking account of an indicator of 'standard of living' (the more direct reflection of the material circumstances of respondents used in Chapter 6) leads to a large reduction in the relative risk (compare the first and last bars). Given that this indicator is also not perfect for taking account of ethnic differences in socio-economic position (see Table 6.13), such a finding suggests that socio-economic differences, in fact, make a large and key contribution to ethnic inequalities in health.

Indeed, a consistent finding in this study was that making adjustments for socio-economic position using the more sensitive standard of living indicator reduced the relative risk of ethnic minority groups compared with white groups to have an adverse health outcome. This is clearly shown in Figure 7.5, which uses the natural logarithm of the relative risk statistic to compare how risk of ill-health across the eight key dimensions considered here changes for ethnic minority respondents compared with whites, once socio-economic position is partially controlled for using the standard of living indicator. In the figure, a risk equivalent to that for whites is represented by the X-axis (i.e. the value 0), and a figure above this represents a greater risk, while a figure below this a smaller risk. In all but one case, diagnosed heart disease for the Caribbean group, the risk for ethnic minority groups compared with whites is reduced once the socio-economic control has been applied. Not

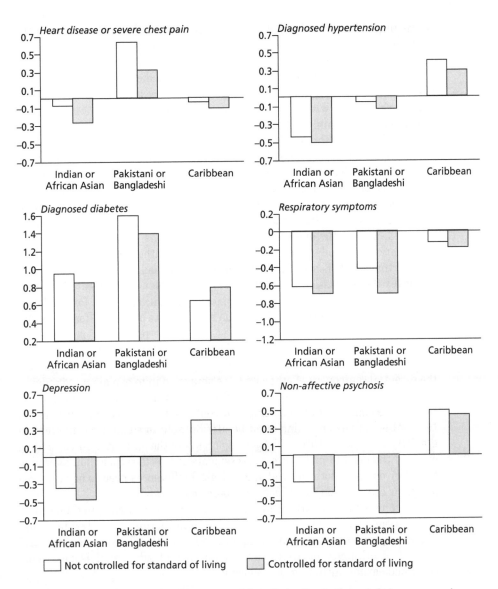

**Figure 7.5  Reduction in the natural log (ln) of relative risk in comparison with white people**

shown in the figure is that in many cases the risk changes from being statistically significantly greater than that for whites to not being so, or from not being different to statistically significantly lower than that for whites.

However, an important message emerging from the analysis presented here and in Chapter 6 is that taking account of socio-economic factors when exploring ethnic inequalities in health is not a straightforward process. It seems likely that few, if any, studies in this area will have the luxury of the depth of relevant information provided by this survey. Consequently, when making comparisons across ethnic groups, researchers should be aware of the limitations of data that only contain crude overall indicators of socio-economic position, such as occupational class or housing tenure and car ownership, that may work well for within-group comparisons (an important task in its own right), but are certainly not adequate for across-group comparisons.

In addition, although the use of an appropriate indicator in making adjustments for socio-economic position reveals important effects, such an approach to analysis and interpretation contains problems because it regards socio-economic position as a confounding factor (McKenzie and Crowcroft, 1996) that needs to be controlled out to reveal the 'true' relationship between ethnicity and health. This results in the importance of socio-economic factors becoming obscured and their explanatory role lost. So, as described above, the presentation of 'standardised' data leaves both the author and reader to assume that all that is left is an 'ethnic/race' effect, be that cultural or genetic. Again, this gives the impression that different types of explanation operate for ethnic minority groups compared with the general population. While for the latter factors relating to socio-economic position are shown to be crucial, for the former they are not visible, so differences are assumed to be related to some aspect of ethnicity or 'race', even though, as shown here, socio-economic factors are important determinants of health for all groups. This allows a theory regarding the essential component of ethnicity to be smuggled in to explain a redundancy in a model that claims to, but cannot, fully account for socio-economic factors. Indeed, the claim that after attempts to 'control out' socio-economic factors the residual effect that remains must be attributable to something inherent in ethnicity – such as culture or biology – ignores both the difficulties in 'controlling out' and the need to make direct assessments of effects rather than assuming that they operate. Both cultural and biological differences need to be measured and their contribution to differences in outcome assessed.

Here it is also important to remember that, as well as being imperfect, socio-economic indicators do not account for other forms of disadvantage that might play some role in ethnic inequalities in health. That is, the structural context of ethnicity needs to cover a number of additional issues, some described earlier, including the following.

1   A lifetime perspective: differences are likely to be a consequence of a lifetime accumulation of disadvantage (Davey Smith et al., 1997), which may be particularly important for migrants who will have been through a number of life-course transitions, and whose childhood might have involved significant deprivation.

2   Living in a racist society: in addition to direct experiences of racism, ethnic minority people know that they are disadvantaged and excluded compared with others, and hence have a clear perception of their relative disadvantage. This sense of relative disadvantage, as Wilkinson (1996)

has argued, may well have a significant impact on health. And there is growing evidence on the relationship between experiences of racism and health. Benzeval et al. (1992) demonstrated that experiencing racial harassment was significantly associated with reported acute illness, although, the Fourth National Survey showed that variations across ethnic minority groups in the reported experiences of racial harassment did not match those for health (Modood et al., 1997) – for example, Bangladeshi people, who had the poorest health, were less likely than African Asian and Chinese people, who had the best health, to report that they had been racially harassed. Karlsen and Nazroo (2001a) have used these data to show that both the experience of racist acts and perceptions of racial discrimination in society are related to poorer health across a variety of outcomes for ethnic minority people. However, the processes that link such perceptions and experiences with poorer health outcomes may not be straightforward. For example, studies in the US have shown that Black Americans who report and challenge racial harassment and discrimination have lower blood pressure than those who say they would tolerate discrimination and do not report experiencing it (Krieger, 1990; Krieger and Sidney, 1996). The authors suggest that, in the case of hypertension at least, the negative health effect is a consequence of internalised anger, which would be more likely among those who experience, but do not report, racial harassment.

3   Ecological effects: ethnic minority people are concentrated in particular geographical locations that are quite different from those populated by the white majority (Owen, 1994a) and there is a growing body of work suggesting that the environmental circumstances may have a direct impact on health over and above individual circumstances (Townsend et al., 1988; Macintyre et al., 1993).

One possible interpretation of the Fourth National Survey findings on socio-economic effects is that ethnic inequalities in health can be reduced to structural, or specifically socio-economic, disadvantage, a position that has been supported by a number of commentators in the field and that raises questions about the legitimacy of using ethnicity as an explanatory variable (Navarro, 1990; Sheldon and Parker, 1992). This potentially reduces ethnicity to class and shifts the focus to a concern with how racism leads to the disadvantaged socio-economic positions of 'ethnic minority' groups (see Miles's (1989) comments on this in relation to 'race'), a position that needs additional empirical support. Indeed, as I pointed out earlier, others have suggested that regardless of any socio-economic contribution, ethnic inequalities in health cannot be reduced to class, because ethnicity involves far more than this (Hillier and Kelleher, 1996; Kelleher, 1996; Smaje, 1996). And, of course, a similar debate is present in the wider literature on ethnicity. Consequently, it is worth considering how ethnicity might be brought back into the picture.

## Ethnicity as identity

Smaje (1996) has commentated that ethnicity needs to be considered both as identity and as structure. Insofar as ethnic minority status can be equated with various forms of disadvantage, ethnicity is perhaps best viewed as an 'external definition' imposed on ethnic minority people by the majority (Jenkins, 1996). In this sense 'ethnicity' is used to signify the 'Other', allowing the construction and maintenance of boundaries of exclusion and hierarchical relationships. Although most commentators on such a process of signification have emphasised the role of physical characteristics and the ideological notion of 'race', they recognise that this process also involves cultural characteristics (e.g. Miles, 1989: 40; Mason, 1996: 201). So, although the biological and cultural can be analytically separated, the ideological representations of 'race' and 'ethnicity' overlap, both representing notions of the inherent, inevitable and inferior biological and cultural characteristics of signified groups (Miles, 1996). Indeed such a relationship between these two concepts is clearly present in the health field, as the example on CHD previously cited illustrates (Gupta et al., 1995). In terms of understanding ethnic inequalities in health, this leads to a focus on the process and origins of 'ethnic' signification (perhaps located in the wider demands of capitalism (Miles, 1989)), how this leads to the disadvantaged position of ethnic minority groups, and the links between that (material) disadvantage and poor health.

In terms of ethnic identity, however, others have argued that underlying the 'racist categorisation' imposed on ethnic minority groups lie 'real collectivities, common and distinctive forms of thinking and behaviour, of language, custom, religion and so on; not just modes of oppression but modes of being' (Modood 1996: 95). This is the 'internal definition' where individuals and groups establish their own identity (Jenkins, 1996). To emphasise this point, some have attempted to draw an ideological distinction between the notions of 'race' and 'ethnicity'. While the former is a boundary of exclusion imposed on a minority group, the latter is a boundary of inclusion, providing a sense of identity and access to social resources. So relations between ethnic groups 'are not necessarily hierarchical, exploitative and conflictual' (Jenkins, 1996: 71). In addition, Modood argues, in the context of his analysis and interpretation of some of the data from this study, that ethnic identity provides a political resource:

> Ethnic identity, like gender and sexuality, has become politicised and for some people has become a primary focus of their politics. There is an ethnic assertiveness, arising out of the feelings of not being respected or lacking access to public space, consisting of counterposing 'positive' images against traditional or dominant stereotypes. It is a politics of projecting identities in order to challenge existing power relations; of seeking not just toleration for ethnic difference but also public acknowledgement, resources and representation (1997: 290).

In this sense a politicised and mobilised ethnic identity can be construed as a new social movement (Scott, 1990) occurring in a vacuum provided by the disappearance of a class-based politics (Gilroy, 1987).

In Chapter 1 it was pointed out that it is important to recognise that this notion of ethnicity is also some considerable distance from the immutable and reified elements of 'race' or a decontexualised identity. Briefly, it is suggested that ethnic identity cannot be considered as fixed, because culture is not an autonomous and static feature in an individual's life. Cultural traditions are historically located; they occur within particular contexts and change over time, place and person. In addition, ethnicity is only one element of identity, whose significance depends on the context within which the individual finds him/herself. For example, gender and class are also important and in certain situations may be more important. The implication is that there are a range of identities that come into play in different contexts and that identity should be regarded as neither secure nor coherent (Hall, 1992; Hillier and Kelleher, 1996; Kelleher, 1996; Smaje, 1996; Ahmad, 1999).

This conception of ethnic identity promises exciting new avenues to follow in the exploration of the relationship between ethnicity and health. Ethnic identity as a source of pride and political power provides an interesting contrast to ethnicity as a sense of discrimination and relative disadvantage, a contrast which could be of great relevance to Wilkinson's (1996) arguments on the relationship between relative deprivation and health. Indeed, there is evidence to suggest that the concentration of ethnic minority groups in particular locations is protective of health (Halpern, 1993; Smaje, 1995a; Halpern and Nazroo, 1999), perhaps because this allows the development of a community with a strong ethnic identity that enhances social support and reduces the sense of alienation. Such a conception of ethnic identity also allows a contextualised culture to be brought into view. Identification with cultural traditions that may be both harmful and, now we can separate ethnicity from the outsiders' negative definition, beneficial to health, are of obvious importance to health promotion.

However, the fluid and contextual nature of ethnic identity, and the potential competition between multiple identities, make this field of enquiry highly complex. For example, Ahmad's (1995) suggestion that we should research the relationship between ethnicity and health with the contextual nature of ethnicity explicitly in mind presents serious methodological problems, as illustrated by Hahn and Stroup's (1994) suggestions that 'standard scientific criteria' may not apply to the measurement of ethnicity, and fluid ethnic boundaries mean 'fuzzy logic' might apply. Such work is also in its infancy, with virtually no empirical work being undertaken. One unique example used data from the Fourth National Survey to examine the dimensions of ethnic identity and how they were related to health, but failed to find an association between type and strength of ethnic identity and health, despite an apparent robustness in its assessment of ethnic identity (Karlsen and Nazroo, 2001b).

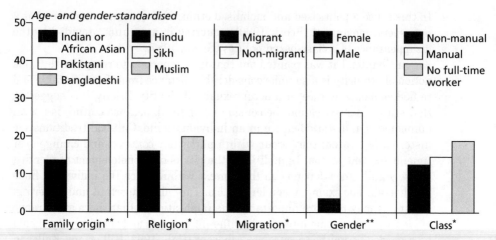

* p < 0.01
** p < 0.001
1 Indians or African Asians only for the religion panel

**Figure 7.6   Smoking by ethnicity, gender and class – South Asians only[1]**

The level of complexity in attempting to unpack identity and structural effects can be illustrated by data from earlier chapters. Figure 7.6 shows how rates of smoking – presumably at least partly a culturally related practice – vary according to a number of criteria. For simplicity's sake, only those with South Asian family origins are included.

The first section of the figure shows that smoking was related to a broadly defined ethnic background. This impression of cultural variation is confirmed if the data are analysed by religion rather than country of family origin (for the Indian or African Asian respondents only). The second section of the figure shows that Sikhs have very low rates of smoking, while Muslims have high rates. The next section of the figure suggests that these elements of culture are not stable. Those who migrated to Britain aged 11 or older (described as migrants in the figure) reported lower rates of smoking, suggesting that this behaviour is related to differences in the cultural context of migrants' and non-migrants' childhoods. This emphasises the need to contextualise ethnic identity to capture its fluid nature, a need that is further emphasised by both the fourth and final sections of the figure. The fourth section shows that gender is also strongly related to smoking, so both ethnic and gender identities need to be considered together. The final section shows that class is also important. Continuing in the vein of the rest of this paragraph, it would make sense to suggest that this has something to do with a class identity, but class is also an indicator of material circumstances and these may play a more important role in predicting smoking. This possibility forces us to reflect back on the interpretation of the other sections of the figure, because they also represent more than just a self-adopted and asserted culture or identity. They correlate with both socio-economic position and externally imposed identities. Here the need for data that go far beyond what we currently have available, as Ahmad (1995) has recommended, becomes very apparent.

## CONCLUSION

I have suggested that to understand the relationship between ethnicity and health we need to theorise ethnicity adequately, and that this involves recognising ethnicity as both structure and identity. When addressing the ontological status of ethnicity, it appears to be important to consider it as a product of social structures, perhaps seeing racial and ethnic categorisation as a product of racism, as Miles (1989) argues, though not necessarily viewing such processes as entirely economically determined. However, it is also important to recognise the role of agency in the production of ethnicity, to view it as a product of social action, and to address the dialectic between agency and structure. Empirically addressing issues relating to ethnic identity, particularly in a quantitative survey, is not straightforward (Ahmad, 1999). But extending the empirical exploration of the relationship between ethnic identity, structure and health inequalities is an important next step, begun by Karlsen and Nazroo's (2001a and 2001b) analyses of the ethnic identity and racism data contained in the Fourth National Survey.

Nevertheless, the evidence presented in this volume provides strong support for a structural–material explanation for ethnic inequalities in health. And, insofar as ethnic differences in health can be seen as a consequence of class inequalities, the discussion so far indicates that work on the relationship between ethnicity and health has the potential to be at the leading edge of inequalities in health research. In terms of the cluster of competing and complementary explanations for class inequalities in health, ethnic background is strongly related to most. There is variation in the class position of different ethnic minority and majority groups, and this is reflected in differing levels and types of material disadvantage. Ethnic minority groups are discriminated against and recognise themselves as disadvantaged. This disadvantage not only occurs in the form of a failure to achieve the full potential of economic success, but also in everyday exclusion from elements of white, mainstream society. Consequently, there is the potential to explore the psychological, as well as material, consequences of disadvantage. Ethnic minority people are concentrated in particular geographical locations and these locations have specific attributes that should allow us to explore both the extent and the nature of an ecological contribution to inequalities in health. Migrant ethnic minority people have been through a number of life-course transitions, some of which would be related to changes in material resources, others to changes in social networks and position in the social hierarchy. Exploring ethnicity also has the potential to allow an examination of the relationship between lifestyle and health and how this might contribute to inequalities. In particular it should allow a dynamic exploration of culture and the relationship between culture, context and class. There are important differences in the social position and expectations of women in different ethnic groups, allowing us to explore issues relating to gender inequalities. And, of course, there are purported differences in the genetic make-up of different ethnic groups.

In terms of methodological issues, exploring ethnic inequalities in health could help resolve a number of problems. Such work relies on indicators of health that are valid across different ethnic groups. Exposing the extent to which the validity of health assessments might vary across ethnic groups raises questions that are applicable to other forms of comparison, such as class and gender. The difficulty of finding indicators of socio-economic position that operate consistently across ethnic groups provides an impetus to be clear about what we mean by the concept of 'class' in this research (Scambler and Higgs, 1999), and how this might apply to other forms of social division, such as gender. And operationalising a concept of ethnicity should make us focus on what we mean by ethnicity and which dimensions of ethnicity might be relevant to inequalities in health.

However, it is worth stepping back for a moment (at least) to reconsider our motives for undertaking work on inequalities in health. In terms of ethnic inequalities in health, I have suggested that motives for the work are related to competing desires to expose the extent and consequences of wider social inequalities, and to uncover aetiological processes, and I have argued that the latter approach has great potential for racialising inequalities in health (Nazroo, 1997c and 1999). Although at first sight it seems that inequalities in health research are very much concerned with the former, a reconsideration of the preceding elements of this section might suggest otherwise. The tight focus on the pathways that lead from disadvantage to poor health should contribute greatly to our understanding of aetiology, particularly if we meet the requirement that material causes of inequalities in health must be biologically plausible. And there is no reason why such pathways should be identical for different health outcomes. This focus produces an exclusive concern with inequalities *in health* as the adverse outcome, and how the complex pathways leading to this outcome can be understood and broken. The root cause, wider social inequalities, becomes obscured from view. The policy implications of this are clear: the more difficult and dramatic interventions to address social inequalities can continue to be avoided and health promotion can focus on improving our understanding of pathways and designing interventions along them. Inequalities in health become a problem requiring technical interventions tailored to individual diseases and individual circumstances; they become a problem for individuals rather than a reflection of social malaise. Williams et al.'s comments in this regard are worth citing:

There is a temptation to focus on identified risk factors as the focal point for intervention efforts. In contrast, we indicate that the macrosocial factors and racism are the basic causes of racial differences in health. The risk factors and resources are the surface causes, the current intervening mechanisms. These may change, but as long as the basic causes remain operative, the modification of surface causes alone will only lead to the emergence of new intervening mechanisms to maintain the same outcome (1994: 36).

We need to remember that we are concerned with (ethnic) inequalities in health because they are a component and a consequence of an inequitable capitalist society, and it is this that needs to be directly addressed.

# References

Adebimpe, V.R. (1994) 'Race, racism, and epidemiological surveys', *Hospital and Community Psychiatry*, vol. 45, no. 1, pp. 27–31

Ahmad, W. (1995) 'Review article: "Race" and health', *Sociology of Health and Illness*, vol. 17, no. 3, pp. 418–29

Ahmad, W. (1999) 'Ethnic statistics: better than nothing or worse than nothing?'. In D. Dorling and S. Simpson (eds) *Statistics in Society: The Arithmetic of Politics*. London: Arnold

Ahmad, W., Sheldon, T. and Stuart, O. (eds) (1996) *Ethnicity and Health: Reviews of the Literature and Guidance for Purchasers in the Areas of Cardiovascular Disease, Mental Health and Haemoglobinopathies*. York: University of York

Ahmad, W.I.U. (1993a) *'Race' and Health in Contemporary Britain*. Buckingham: Open University Press

Ahmad, W.I.U. (1993b) 'Making black people sick: "race", ideology and health research'. In W.I.U. Ahmad (ed.) *'Race' and Health in Contemporary Britain*. Buckingham: Open University Press

Ahmad, W.I.U. (1996) 'The trouble with culture'. In D. Kelleher and S. Hillier (eds) *Researching Cultural Differences in Health*, London: Routledge

Ahmad, W.I.U., Kernohan, E.E.M. and Baker, M.R. (1989) 'Influence of ethnicity and unemployment on the perceived health of a sample of general practice attenders', *Community Medicine*, vol. 11, no. 2, pp. 148–56

Ahmad, W.I.U. and Sheldon, T. (1993) '"Race" and statistics'. In M. Hammersley (ed.) *Social Research: Philosophy, Politics and Practice*. London: Sage

American Psychiatric Association (1995) *Diagnostic and Statistical Manual IV*. Washington DC: APA

Andrews, A. and Jewson, N. (1993) 'Ethnicity and infant deaths: the implications of recent statistical evidence for materialist explanations', *Sociology of Health and Illness*, vol. 15, no. 2, pp. 137–56

Anionwu, E. (1993) 'Sickle cell and thalassaemia: community experiences and official response'. In W.I.U. Ahmad (ed.) *'Race' and Health in Contemporary Britain*. Buckingham: Open University Press

Arber, S. (1990) 'Opening the 'black' box: understanding inequalities in women's health'. In P. Abbott and G. Payne (eds) *New Directions in the Sociology of Health*. Brighton: Falmer Press

Aspinall, P. (1995) 'Department of Health's requirement for mandatory collection of data on ethnic group of inpatients', *British Medical Journal*, vol. 311, pp. 1006–9

Atkin, K. and Ahmad, W.I.U. (1996) 'Ethnicity and caring for a disabled child: the case of children with sickle cell or thalassaemia', *British Journal of Social Work*, vol. 26, pp. 755–75

Badger, F., Atkin, K. and Griffiths, R. (1989) 'Why don't general practitioners refer their disabled Asian patients to district nurses?', *Health Trends*, vol. 21, pp. 31–2

Bagley, C. (1971) 'The social aetiology of schizophrenia in immigrant groups', *International Journal of Social Psychiatry*, vol. 17, pp. 292–304

Bagley, C. (1995) 'A plea for ignoring race and including insured status in American research reports on social science and medicine', *Social Science and Medicine*, vol. 40, no. 8, pp. 1017–19

Balarajan, R. (1991) 'Ethnic differences in mortality from ischaemic heart disease and cerebrovascular disease in England and Wales', *British Medical Journal*, vol. 302, pp. 560–4

Balarajan, R. (1996) 'Ethnicity and variations in the nation's health', *Health Trends*, vol. 27, no. 4, pp. 114–19

Balarajan, R. and Bulusu, L. (1990) 'Mortality among immigrants in England and Wales, 1979–83'. In M. Britton (ed.) *Mortality and Geography: A Review in the Mid-1980s, England and Wales*. London: OPCS

Balarajan, R., Bulusu, L., Adelstein, A.M. and Shukla, V. (1984) 'Patterns of mortality among migrants to England and Wales from the Indian subcontinent', *British Medical Journal*, vol. 289, pp. 1185–7

Balarajan, R. and Soni Raleigh, V. (1993) *The Health of the Nation: Ethnicity and Health*. London: Department of Health

Balarajan, R. and Soni Raleigh, V. (1995) *Ethnicity and Health in England*, London: HMSO

Barker, D. (1991) 'The foetal and infant origins of inequalities in health in Britain', *Journal of Public Health Medicine*, vol. 13, pp. 64–8

Barot, R. (ed.) (1996) *The Racism Problematic: Contemporary Sociological Debates on Race and Ethnicity*, Lewiston: The Edwin Mellen Press

Bartley, M. (1994) 'Unemployment and ill health: understanding the relationship', *Journal of Epidemiology and Community Health*, vol. 48, pp. 333–7

Bartley, M., Montgomery, S., Cook, D. and Wadsworth, M. (1996) 'Health and work insecurity in young men'. In D. Blane, E. Brunner and R. Wilkinson (eds) *Health and Social Organisation*. London: Routledge

Battle, R.M., Pathak, D., Humble, C.G., Key, C.R., Vanatta, P.R., Hill, R.B. and Anderson, R.E. (1987) 'Factors influencing discrepancies between premortem and postmortem diagnoses', *Journal of the American Medical Association*, vol. 258, no. 3, pp. 339–44

Bebbington, P. (1996) 'The origins of sex differences in depressive disorder: bridging the gap', *International Review of Psychiatry*, vol. 8, pp. 295–332

Bebbington, P.E., Feeney, S.T., Flannigan, C.B., Glover, G.R., Lewis, S.W and Wing, J.K. (1994) 'Inner London collaborative audit of admisssions in two health districts. II: Ethnicity and the use of the Mental Health Act', *British Journal of Psychiatry*, vol. 165, no. 6, pp. 743–9

Bebbington, P. and Nayani, T. (1995) 'The psychosis screening questionnaire', *International Journal of Methods in Psychiatric Research*, vol. 5, pp. 11–19

Beishon, S. and Nazroo, J.Y. (1997) *Coronary Heart Disease: Contrasting the Health Beliefs and Behaviours of South Asian Communities in the UK*. London: Health Education Authority

Ben-Shlomo, Y., White, I.R. and Marmot, M. (1996) 'Does the variation in the socioeconomic characteristics of an area affect mortality?', *British Medical Journal*, vol. 312, pp. 1013–14

Benzeval, M., Judge, K. and Solomon, M. (1992) *The Health Status of Londoners*. London: King's Fund

Benzeval, M., Judge, K. and Whitehead, M. (1995) *Tackling Inequalities in Health: An Agenda for Action*. London: King's Fund

Berthoud, R. (1997) 'Income and standards of living'. In T. Modood, R. Berthoud, J. Lakey, J. Nazroo, P. Smith, S. Virdee and S. Beishon, *Ethnic Minorities in Britain: Diversity and Disadvantage*. London: Policy Studies Institute

Berthoud, R. and Beishon, S. (1997) 'People, families and households'. In T. Modood, R. Berthoud, J. Lakey, J. Nazroo, P. Smith, S. Virdee and S. Beishon, *Ethnic Minorities in Britain: Diversity and Disadvantage*. London: Policy Studies Institute

Bhopal, R. (1997) 'Is research into ethnicity and health racist, unsound, or important science?', *British Medical Journal*, vol. 314, pp. 1751–6

Bhugra, D., Hilwig, M., Hossein, B., Marceau, H., Neehall, J., Leff, J., Mallett, R. and Der, G. (1996) 'First-contact incidence rates of schizophrenia in Trinidad and one-year follow-up', *British Journal of Psychiatry*, vol. 169, pp. 587–92

Bhugra, D., Leff, J., Mallett, R., Der, G., Corridan, B. and Rudge, S. (1997) 'Incidence and outcome of schizophrenia in whites, African-Caribbeans and Asians in London', *Psychological Medicine*, vol. 27, pp. 791–8

Biswas, S. (1990) 'Ethnic differences in self poisoning: a comparative study between an Asian and White adolescent group', *Journal of Adolescence*, vol. 13, pp. 189–93

Blalock, H.M. (1985) *Social Statistics*. Singapore: McGraw-Hill

Blane, D., Bartley, M., Davey Smith, G., Filakti, H., Bethune, A. and Harding, S. (1994) 'Social patterning of medical mortality in youth and early adulthood', *Social Science and Medicine*, vol. 39, no. 3, pp. 361–6

Blane, D., Power, C. and Bartley, M. (1996) 'Illness behaviour and the measurement of class differentials in morbidity', *Journal of the Royal Statistical Society*, vol. 156, no. 1, pp. 77–92

Blaxter, M. (1987) 'Evidence of inequality in health from a national survey', *The Lancet*, vol. 2, no. 8549, pp. 30–3

Blaxter, M. (1990) *Health and Lifestyles*. London: Tavistock/Routledge

Bloor, M.J., Robertson, C. and Samphier, M.L. (1989) 'Occupational status variations in disagreements on the diagnosis of cause of death', *Human Pathology*, vol. 30, pp. 144–8

Bradby, H. (1995) 'Ethnicity: not a black and white issue. A research note', *Sociology of Health and Illness*, vol. 17, no. 3, pp. 405–17

Brown, C. (1984) *Black and White Britain: The Third PSI Survey*, London: Heinemann

Brown, C. and Ritchie, J. (1981) *Focused Enumeration: The Development of a Method for Sampling Ethnic Minority Groups*. London: Policy Studies Institute/SCPR

Cameron, H.M. and McGoogan, E. (1981) 'A prospective study of 1,152 hospital autopsies: I. Inaccuracies in death certification', *Pathology*, vol. 133, pp. 273–83

Carpenter, L. and Brockington, I.F. (1980) 'A study of mental illness in Asians, West Indians and Africans living in Manchester', *British Journal of Psychiatry*, vol. 137, pp. 201–5

Chaturvedi, N. and McKeigue, P. (1994) 'Methods for epidemiological surveys of ethnic minority groups', *Journal of Epidemiology and Community Health*, vol. 48, pp. 107–11

Chaturvedi, N., Rai, H. and Ben-Shlomo, Y. (1997) 'Lay diagnosis and health care seeking behaviour for chest pain in South Asians and Europeans', *Lancet*, vol. 350, pp. 1578–83

Clarke, M., Clayton, D.G., Mason, E.S. and MacVicar, J. (1988) 'Asian mothers' risk factors for perinatal death – the same or different? A 10-year review of Leicestershire perinatal deaths', *British Medical Journal*, vol. 297, pp. 384–87

Cochrane, R. and Bal, S.S. (1989) 'Mental hospital admission rates of immigrants to England: a comparison of 1971 and 1981', *Social Psychiatry and Psychiatric Epidemiology*, vol. 24, pp. 2–11

Cochrane, R. and Sashidharan, S.P. (1996) 'Mental health and ethnic minorities: a review of the literature and implications for services'. In W. Ahmad, T. Sheldon and O. Stuart (eds) *Ethnicity and Health*. York: University of York

Cochrane, R. and Stopes-Roe, M. (1981) 'Psychological symptom levels in Indian immigrants to England – a comparison with native English', *Psychological Medicine*, vol. 11, pp. 319–27

Cole, E., Leavey, G., King, M., Johnson-Sabine, E. and Hoar, A. (1995) 'Pathways to care for patients with a first episode of psychosis: a comparison of ethnic groups', *British Journal of Psychiatry*, vol. 167, pp. 770–6

Coleman, D. and Salt, J. (1996) *Ethnicity in the 1991 Census. Volume 1: Demographic Characteristics of the Ethnic Minority Populations*. London: HMSO

Cooper, J.E., Goodhead, D., Craig, T., Harris, M., Howat, J. and Korer, J. (1987) 'The Incidence of Schizophrenia in Nottingham', *British Journal of Psychiatry*, vol. 151, pp. 619–26

Cruickshank, J., Beevers, D., Osbourne, R., Haynes, J., Corlett, J. and Selby, S. (1980) 'Heart attack, stroke, diabetes, and hypertension in West Indians, Asians and whites in Birmingham, England', *British Medical Journal*, vol. 281, pp. 1108

Cruickshank, J.K., Cooper, J.E., Burnett, M., MacDuff, J. and Drubra, U. (1991) 'Ethnic differences in fasting plasma C-peptide and insulin in relation to glucose tolerance and blood pressure', *Lancet*, vol. 338, pp. 842–7

Daniel, W.W. (1968) *Racial Discrimination in England*. London: Penguin

Davey Smith, G., Bartley, M. and Blane, D. (1990a) 'The Black report on socioeconomic inequalities in health 10 years on', *British Medical Journal*, vol. 301, pp. 373–7

Davey Smith, G., Blane, D. and Bartley, M. (1994) 'Explanations for socio-economic differentials in mortality: evidence from Britain and elsewhere', *European Journal of Public Health*, vol. 4, pp. 131–44

Davey Smith, G., Hart, C., Blane, D., Gillis, C. and Hawthorne, V. (1997) 'Lifetime socioeconomic position and mortality: prospective observational study', *British Medical Journal*, vol. 314, pp. 547–52

Davey Smith, G., Neaton, J.D., Wentworth, D., Stamler, R. and Stamler, J. (1998) 'Mortality differences between black and white men in the USA: contribution of income and other risk factors among men screened for the MRFIT', *The Lancet*, vol. 351, pp. 934–9

Davey Smith, G., Shipley, M.J. and Rose, G. (1990b) 'Magnitude and causes of socioeconomic differentials in mortality: further evidence from the Whitehall study', *Journal of Epidemiology and Community Health*, vol. 44, p. 265

Davey Smith, G., Wentworth, D., Neaton, J.D., Stamler, R. and Stamler, J. (1996) 'Socioeconomic differentials in mortality risk among men screened for the Multiple Risk Factor Intervention Trial: Part II – results for 20,224 black men', *American Journal of Public Health*, vol. 86, pp. 497–504

Davies, S., Modell, B. and Wonke, B. (1993) 'The haemoglobinopathies: impact upon Black and ethnic minority people'. In A. Hopkins and V. Bahl (eds) *Access to Health Care for People from Black and Ethnic Minorities*. London: Royal College of Physicians

Davies, S., Thornicroft, G., Leese, M., Higgingbotham, A. and Phelan, M. (1996) 'Ethnic differences in risk of compulsory psychiatric admission among representative cases of psychosis in London', *British Medical Journal*, vol. 312, pp. 533–7

Dean, G., Walsh, D., Downing, H., and Shelley, E. (1981) 'First admissions of native-born and immigrants to psychiatric hospitals in south-east England 1976', *British Journal of Psychiatry*, vol. 139, pp. 506–12

Department of Health (1992) *The Health of the Nation: A Strategy for Health in England*. London: HMSO

Department of Health (1995) *Variations in Health. What Can the Department of Health and the NHS Do?* London: Department of Health

Donovan, J. (1984) 'Ethnicity and health: a research review', *Social Science and Medicine*, vol. 19, no. 7, pp. 663–70

Drever, F. and Whitehead, M. (1997) *Health Inequalities: Decennial supplement No. 15*, London: The Stationery Office

Dunnell, K. (1993) *Sources and Nature of Ethnic Health Data.* London: North East and North West Thames RHA

Erens, B., Primatesta, P. and Prior, G. (eds) (2001) *Health Survey for England: The Health of Minority Ethnic Groups.* London: The Stationery Office

Fenton, S., Hughes, A. and Hine, C. (1995) 'Self-assessed health, economic status and ethnic origin', *New Community*, vol. 21, no. 1, pp. 55–68

Fenton, S. and Sadiq-Sangster, A. (1996) 'Culture, relativism and the expression of mental distress: South Asian women in Britain', *Sociology of Health and Illness*, vol. 18, no. 1, pp. 66–85

Fox, K. and Shapiro, L. (1988) 'Heart disease in Asians in Britain', *British Medical Journal*, vol. 297, pp. 311–12

Gatrell, A. (1997) 'Structures of geographical and social space and their consequences for human health', *Geografiska Annaler*, vol. 79, no. 3, pp. 141–51

Gilliam, S.J., Jarman, B., White, P. and Law, R. (1989) 'Ethnic differences in consultation rates in urban general practice', *British Medical Journal*, vol. 299, pp. 953–7

Gilroy, P. (1987) *There Ain't No Black in the Union Jack: The Cultural Politics of Race and Nation.* London: Hutchinson

Glover, G.R. (1989) 'Why is there a high rate of schizophrenia in British Caribbeans?', *British Journal of Hospital Medicine*, vol. 42, pp. 48–51

Gordon, T. (1982) 'Further mortality experience among Japanese Americans', *Public Health Reports*, vol. 97, pp. 973–84

Gould, M.I. and Jones, K. (1996) 'Analyzing perceived limiting long-term illness using UK census microdata', *Social Science and Medicine*, vol. 42, no. 6, pp. 857–69

Gupta, R., Gupta, V.P. and Ahluwalia, N.S. (1994) 'Educational status, coronary heart disease, and coronary risk factor prevalence in a rural population of India', *British Medical Journal*, vol. 309, pp. 1332–6

Gupta, S., de Belder, A. and O'Hughes, L. (1995) 'Avoiding premature coronary deaths in Asians in Britain: spend now on prevention or pay later for treatment', *British Medical Journal*, vol. 311, pp. 1035–6

Hahn, R.A. and Stroup, D.F. (1994) 'Race and ethnicity in public health surveillance: criteria for the scientific use of social categories', *Public Health Reports*, vol. 109, no. 1, pp. 7–15

Hall, S. (1992) 'The question of cultural identity'. In S. Hall, D. Held and T. McGrew (eds) *Modernity and its Futures.* Cambridge: Polity

Halpern, D. (1993) 'Minorities and mental health', *Social Science and Medicine*, vol. 36, no. 5, pp. 597–607

Halpern, D. and Nazroo, J. (2000) 'The ethnic density effect: results from a national community survey of England and Wales', *The International Journal of Social Psychiatry*, vol. 46, no. 1, pp. 34–46

Handy, S., Chithiramohan, R.N., Ballard, C.G. and Silveira, W.R. (1991) 'Ethnic differences in adolescent self-poisoning: a comparison of Asian and Caucasian groups', *Journal of Adolescence*, vol. 14, pp. 157–62

Harding, S. and Maxwell, R. (1997) 'Differences in the mortality of migrants'. In Drever, F. and Whitehead, M. (eds) *Health Inequalities: Decennial Supplement Series DS no. 15*, London: The Stationery Office

Harrison, G., Holton, A., Neilson, D., Owens, D., Boot, D. and Cooper, J. (1989) 'Severe mental disorder in Afro-Caribbean patients: some social, demographic and service factors', *Psychological Medicine*, vol. 19, pp. 683–96

Harrison, G., Owens, D., Holton, A., Neilson, D. and Boot, D. (1988) 'A prospective study of severe mental disorder in Afro-Caribbean patients', *Psychological Medicine*, vol. 18, pp. 643–57

Harvey, I., Williams, P., McGuffin, P. and Toone, B.K. (1990) 'The functional psychoses in Afro-Caribbeans', *British Journal of Psychiatry*, vol. 157, pp. 515–22

Haynes, R. (1991) 'Inequalities in health and health service use: evidence from the General Household Survey', *Social Science and Medicine*, vol. 33, no. 4, pp. 361–8

Heath, A. and Ridge, J. (1983) 'Social mobility of ethnic minorities', *Journal of Biosocial Science, Supplement*, vol. 8, pp. 169–84

Hickling, F.W. (1991) 'Psychiatric hospital admission rates in Jamaica', *British Journal of Psychiatry*, vol. 159, pp. 817–821

Hickling, F.W. and Rodgers-Johnson, P. (1995) 'The incidence of first contact schizophrenia in Jamaica', *British Journal of Psychiatry*, vol. 167, pp. 193–6

Hill, S.A. (1994) *Sickle Cell Disease in Low Income Families*. Philadelphia, PA: Temple University Press

Hillier, S. and Kelleher, D. (1996) 'Considering culture, ethnicity and the politics of health'. In D. Kelleher and S. Hillier (eds) *Researching Cultural Differences in Health*. London: Routledge

Howlett, B., Ahmad, W. and Murray, R. (1992) 'An exploration of white, Asian and Afro-Caribbean people's concepts of health and illness causation', *New Community*, vol. 18, no. 2, pp. 7–13

Hull, D. (1979) 'Migration, adaptation and illness', *Social Science and Medicine*, vol. 13, pp. 25–36

Humphrey, K. and Carr-Hill, R. (1991) 'Area variations in health outcomes: artefact or ecology', *International Journal of Epidemiology*, vol. 20, no. 1, pp. 251–8

Independent Inquiry into Inequalities in Health (1998) *Report*. London: The Stationery Office

Jadhav, S. (1996) 'The cultural origins of Western depression', *International Journal of Social Psychiatry*, vol. 42, no. 4, pp. 269–86

Jenkins, R. (1986) *Racism in Recruitment*. Cambridge: Cambridge University Press

Jenkins, R. (1996) '"Us" and "them": ethnicity, racism and ideology'. In R. Barot (ed.) *The Racism Problematic: Contemporary Sociological Debates on Race and Ethnicity*. Lewiston: The Edwin Mellen Press

Johnson, M.R.D., Owen D. and Blackburn C. (2000) *Black and Ethnic Minority Groups in England, The Second Health and Lifestyles Survey*. London: Health Education Authority

Joint Committee of the Royal Colleges of Physicians and Pathologists (1982) 'Medical aspects of death certification', *Journal of the Royal College of Physicians*, vol. 16, pp. 205–18

Karlsen, S. and Nazroo, J.Y. (2001a) 'The relationship between racial discrimination, social class and health among ethnic minority groups', *American Journal of Public Health*, in press

Karlsen, S. and Nazroo, J.Y. (2001b) 'Agency and structure: the impact of ethnic identity and racism on the health of ethnic minority people', *Sociology of Health and Illness*, in press

Karmi, G., Abdulrahim, D., Pierpoint, T. and McKeigue, P. (1994) *Suicide among Ethnic Minorities and Refugees in the UK*. London: NE and NW Thames Regional Health Authorities

Karn, V. (ed.) (1997) *Ethnicity in the 1991 Census. Volume 4: Employment, Education and Housing among the Ethnic Minority Populations of Britain*. London: HMSO

Kaufman, J.S., Cooper, R.S. and McGee, D.L. (1997) 'Socioeconomic status and health in blacks and whites: the problem of residual confounding and the resiliency of race', *Epidemiology*, vol. 8, no. 6, pp. 621–8

Kaufman, J.S., Long, A.E., Liao, Y., Cooper, R.S. and McGee, D.L. (1998) 'The relation between income and mortality in US Blacks and Whites', *Epidemiology*, vol. 9, no. 2, pp. 147–55

Kelleher, D. (1996) 'A defence of the use of the terms "ethnicity" and "culture"'. In D. Kelleher and S. Hillier (eds) *Researching Cultural Differences in Health*. London: Routledge

Kelleher, D. and Hillier, S. (eds) (1996) *Researching Cultural Differences in Health*. London: Routledge

Khan, V. (1979) *Minority Families in Britain: Support and Stress.* London: Macmillan

King, M., Coker, E., Leavey, G., Hoare, A. and Johnson-Sabine, E. (1994) 'Incidence of psychotic illness in London: comparison of ethnic groups', *British Medical Journal*, vol. 309, pp. 1115–9

Kleinman, A. (1987) 'Anthropology and psychiatry: the role of culture in cross-cultural research on illness', *British Journal of Psychiatry*, vol. 151, pp. 447–54

Knight, T.M., Smith, Z., Whittles, A., Sahotaa, P., Lockton, J.A., Hogg, G., Bedford, A., Toop, M., (1992) 'Insulin resistance, diabetes, and risk markers for ischaemic heart disease in Asian men and non-Asian men in Bradford', *British Heart Journal*, vol. 67, pp. 343–50

Krause, I. (1989) 'Sinking heart: a Punjabi communication of distress', *Social Science and Medicine*, vol. 29, no. 4, pp. 563–75

Krieger, N. (1990) 'Racial and gender discrimination: risk factors for high blood pressure?', *Social Science and Medicine*, vol. 30, pp. 1273–81

Krieger, N. (1994) 'Epidemiology and the web of causation: has anyone seen the spider?', *Social Science and Medicine*, vol. 39, no. 7, pp. 887–903

Krieger, N. and Sidney, S. (1996) 'Racial discrimination and blood pressure: the CARDIA study of young black and white adults', *American Journal of Public Health*, vol. 86, no. 10, pp. 1370–8

Kuh, D.J.L. and Wadsworth, M.E.J. (1993) 'Physical health status at 36 years in a British national birth cohort', *Social Science and Medicine*, vol. 37, no. 7, pp. 905–16

Lear, J.T., Lawrence, I.G., Burden, A.C. and Pohl, J.E. (1994a) 'A comparison of stress test referral rates and outcome between Asians and Europeans', *Journal of the Royal Society of Medicine*, vol. 87, no. 11, pp. 661–2

Lear, J.T., Lawrence, I.G., Pohl, J.E. and Burden, A.C. (1994b) 'Myocardial infarction and thrombolysis: a comparison of the Indian and European populations on a coronary care unit', *Journal of the Royal College of Physicians*, vol. 28, no. 2, pp. 143–7

Lewis, G., Pelosi, A.J., Araya, R. and Dunn, G. (1992) 'Measuring psychiatric disorder in the community: a standard assessment for use by lay interviewers', *Psychological Medicine*, vol. 22, pp. 465–86

Lillie-Blanton, M. and Laveist, T. (1996) 'Race/ethnicity, the social environment, and health', *Social Science and Medicine*, vol. 43, no. 1, pp. 83–91

Lipsedge, M. (1993) 'Mental health: access to care for black and ethnic minority people'. In A. Hopkins and V. Bahl (eds) *Access to Health Care for People from Black and Ethnic Minorities.* London: Royal College of Physicians

Littlewood, R. (1992) 'Psychiatric diagnosis and racial bias: empirical and interpretative approaches', *Social Science and Medicine*, vol. 34, no. 2, pp. 141–9

Littlewood, R. and Lipsedge, M. (1981) 'Acute psychotic reactions in Caribbean born patients', *Psychological Medicine*, vol. 11, pp. 303–18

Littlewood, R. and Lipsedge, M. (1988) 'Psychiatric illness among British Afro-Caribbeans', *British Medical Journal*, vol. 296, pp. 950–1

Lloyd, K. (1993) 'Depression and anxiety among Afro-Caribbean general practice attenders in Britain', *International Journal of Social Psychiatry*, vol. 39, pp. 1–9

Lowy, A.G.J., Woods, K.L. and Botha, J.L. (1991) 'The effects of demographic shift on coronary heart disease mortality in a large immigrant population at high risk', *Journal of Public Health Medicine*, vol. 13, pp. 276–80

Lundeberg, O. (1991) 'Causal explanations for class inequality in health – an empirical analysis', *Social Science and Medicine*, vol. 32, no. 4, pp. 385–93

MacCarthy, B. and Craissati, J. (1989) 'Ethnic differences in response to adversity: a community sample of Bangladeshis and their indigenous neighbours', *Social Psychiatry and Psychiatric Epidemiology*, vol. 24, pp. 196–201

McGovern, D. and Cope, R. (1987) 'First psychiatric admission rates of first and second generation Afro-Caribbeans', *Social Psychiatry*, vol. 22, pp. 139–49

McGovern, D., Hemmings, P., Cope, R. and Lowerson, A. (1994) 'Long-term follow-up of young Afro-Caribbean Britons and white Britons with a first admission diagnosis of schizophrenia', *Social Psychiatry and Psychiatric Epidemiology*, vol. 29, pp. 8–19

Macintyre, S. (1997) 'The Black Report and beyond: what are the issues?', *Social Science and Medicine*, vol. 44, no. 6, pp. 723–745

Macintyre, S., Maciver, S. and Soomans, A. (1993) 'Area, class and health: should we be focusing on places or people?', *Journal of Social Policy*, vol. 22, no. 2, pp. 213–34

McKeigue, P. (1992) 'Coronary heart disease in Indians, Pakistanis and Bangladeshis: aetiology and possibilities for prevention', *British Heart Journal*, vol. 67, pp. 341–42

McKeigue, P. (1993) *Coronary Heart Disease and Diabetes in South Asians*. London: North East and North West Thames Regional Health Authorities

McKeigue, P. and Marmot, M. (1988) 'Mortality from coronary heart disease in Asian communities in London', *British Medical Journal*, vol. 297, p. 903

McKeigue, P., Marmot, M., Syndercombe Court, Y., Cottier, D., Rahman, S. and Riermersma, R. (1988) 'Diabetes, hyperinsulinaemia, and coronary risk factors in Bangladeshis in East London', *British Heart Journal*, vol. 60, pp. 390–6

McKeigue, P., Miller, G. and Marmot, M. (1989) 'Coronary heart disease in South Asians overseas: a review', *Journal of Clinical Epidemiology*, vol. 42, no. 7, pp. 597–609

McKeigue, P. and Sevak, L. (1994) *Coronary Heart Disease in South Asian Communities*. London: Health Education Authority

McKeigue, P.M., Shah, B. and Marmot, M.G. (1991) 'Relation of central obesity and insulin resistance with high diabetes prevalence and cardiovascular risk in South Asians', *Lancet*, vol. 337, pp. 382–6

Mackenback, J.P., Looman, C.W. and van der Meer, J.B. (1996) 'Differences in the misreporting of chronic conditions by level of education: the effect on inequalities in prevalence rates', *American Journal of Public Health*, vol. 86, no. 5, pp. 706–11

McKenney, N.R. and Bennett, C.E. (1994) 'Issues regarding data on race and ethnicity: the census bureau experience', *Public Health Reports*, vol. 109, no. 1, pp. 16–25

McKenzie, K. and Crowcroft, N. (1994) 'Race, ethnicity, culture, and science', *British Medical Journal*, vol. 309, pp. 286–7

McKenzie, K. and Crowcroft, N. (1996) 'Describing race, ethnicity, and culture in medical research', *British Medical Research*, vol. 312, p. 1054

McKenzie, K., van Os, J., Fahy, T., Jones, P., Harvey, I., Toone, B. and Murray, R. (1995) 'Psychosis with good prognosis in Afro-Caribbean people now living in the United Kingdom', *British Medical Journal*, vol. 311, pp. 1325–8

McKinlay, J.B. (1996) 'Some contributions from the social system to gender inequalities in heart disease', *Journal of Health and Social Behavior*, vol. 37, pp. 1–26

Markowe, H. (1993) 'The work of the Central Health Monitoring Unit in the Department of Health (England)', *Journal of Epidemiology and Community Health*, vol. 47, pp. 6–9

Marmot, M.G., Adelstein, A.M., Bulusu, L. and OPCS (1984) *Immigrant Mortality in England and Wales 1970–78: Causes of Death by Country of Birth*. London: HMSO

Mason, D. (1996) 'Some reflections on the sociology of race and racism'. In R. Barot (ed.) *The Racism Problematic: Contemporary Sociological Debates on Race and Ethnicity*. Lewiston: The Edwin Mellen Press

Mather, H.M. and Keen, H. (1985) 'The Southall diabetes survey: prevalence of known diabetes in Asians and Europeans', *British Medical Journal*, vol. 291, pp. 1081–4

Mather, H.M., Verma, N.P.S., Mehta, S.P., Madhu, S. and Keen, H. (1987) 'The prevalence of known diabetes in Indians in New Delhi and London', *Journal of Medical Association of Thailand*, vol. 70, pp. 54–8

Maxwell, R. and Harding, S. (1998) 'Mortality of migrants from outside England and Wales by marital status', *Population Trends*, vol. 91, pp. 15–22

Meltzer, H., Gill, B., Petticrew, M. and Hinds, K. (1995) *The Prevalence of Psychiatric Morbidity among Adults Living in Private Households*. London: HMSO

Merrill, J. and Owens, J. (1986) 'Ethnic differences in self-poisoning: a comparison of Asian and White groups', *British Journal of Psychiatry*, vol. 148, pp. 708–12

Miles, R. (1989) *Racism*. London: Routledge

Miles, R. (1996) 'Racism and nationalism in the United Kingdom: a view from the periphery'. In R. Barot (ed.) *The Racism Problematic: Contemporary Sociological Debates on Race and Ethnicity*. Lewiston: The Edwin Mellen Press

Modood, T. (1994) 'Political blackness and British Asians', *Sociology*, vol. 28, no. 4, pp. 859–76

Modood, T. (1996) 'If races don't exist, then what does? Racial categorisation and ethnic realities'. In R. Barot (ed.) *The Racism Problematic: Contemporary Sociological Debates on Race and Ethnicity*. Lewiston: The Edwin Mellen Press

Modood, T. (1997a) 'Employment'. In T. Modood, R. Berthoud, J. Lakey, J. Nazroo, P. Smith, S. Virdee and S. Beishon, *Ethnic Minorities in Britain: Diversity and Disadvantage*. London: Policy Studies Institute

Modood, T. (1997b) 'Culture and Identity'. In T. Modood, R. Berthoud, J. Lakey, J. Nazroo, P. Smith, S. Virdee and S. Beishon, *Ethnic Minorities in Britain: Diversity and Disadvantage*. London: Policy Studies Institute

Modood, T. (1998) 'Anti-Essentialism, multiculturalism and the "recognition" of religious groups', *The Journal of Political Philosophy*, vol. 6, no. 4, pp. 378–99

Modood, T., Beishon, S. and Virdee, S. (1994) *Changing Ethnic Identities*. London: Policy Studies Institute

Modood, T., Berthoud, R., Lakey, J., Nazroo, J., Smith, P., Virdee, S. and Beishon, S. (1997) *Ethnic Minorities in Britain: Diversity and Disadvantage*. London: Policy Studies Institute

Morrison, C., Woodward, M., Leslie, W. and Tunstall-Pedoe, H. (1997) 'Effect of socioeconomic group on incidence of, management of, and survival after myocardial infarction and coronary death: analysis of community coronary event register', *British Medical Journal*, vol. 314, pp. 541–6

Mossey, J. and Shapiro, E. (1982) 'Self-rated health: a predictor of mortality among the elderly', *American Journal of Public Health*, vol. 72, pp. 800–8

MRC (Medical Research Council) (1982) *American Thoracic Society News*, vol. 8, pp. 12–16

NACRO Mental Health Advisory Committee (1995) *Mentally Disturbed Prisoners*. London: National Association for the Care and Resettlement of Offenders

Navarro, V. (1990) 'Race or class versus race and class: mortality differentials in the United States', *The Lancet*, vol. 336, pp. 1238–40

Nazroo, J.Y. (1997a) *The Health of Britain's Ethnic Minorities: Findings from a National Survey*. London: Policy Studies Institute

Nazroo, J.Y. (1997b) *Ethnicity and Mental Health: Findings from a National Community Survey*. London: Policy Studies Institute

Nazroo, J.Y. (1997c) 'Why do research on ethnicity and health?', *Share*, no. 18, pp. 5–8

Nazroo, J.Y. (1998) 'Genetic, cultural or socio-economic vulnerability? Explaining ethnic inequalities in health', *Sociology of Health and Illness*, vol. 20, no. 5, pp. 710–30

Nazroo, J.Y. (1999) 'The racialisation of ethnic inequalities in health'. In D. Dorling and S. Simpson (eds) *Statistics in Society: The Arithmetic of Politics*. London: Arnold

Nazroo, J.Y. (in press, 2001) 'South Asians and heart disease: an assessment of the importance of socioeconomic position', *Ethnicity and Disease*, vol. 11, no. 3

Nazroo, J., Becher, H., Kelly, Y. and McMunn, A. (2001) 'Children's Health'. In B.Erens and P. Primatesta (eds) *Health Survey for England: The Health of Minority Ethnic Groups*. London: The Stationery Office

Nazroo, J.Y., Edwards, A.C. and Brown, G.W. (1998) 'Gender differences in the prevalence of depression: artefact, alternative disorders, biology or roles?', *Sociology of Health and Illness*, vol. 20, no. 3, pp. 312–20

Odugbesan, O., Rowe, B., Fletcher, J., Walford, S. and Barnett, A.H. (1989) 'Diabetes in the UK West Indian community: the Wolverhampton study', *Diabetic Medicine*, vol. 9, pp. 641–5

OPS (Office of Population Censuses and Surveys) (1991) *General Household Survey 1989*. London: HMSO

OPS (Office of Population Censuses and Surveys) (1994) *Undercoverage in Great Britain (census user guide no. 58)*. London: HMSO

Owen, D. (1992) *Ethnic Minorities in Great Britain: Settlement Patterns*, National Ethnic Minority Data Archive 1991 Census Statistical Paper no. 1. University of Warwick: Centre for Research in Ethnic Relations

Owen, D. (1993) *Ethnic Minorities in Britain: Age and Gender Structure*, National Ethnic Minority Data Archive 1991 Census Statistical Paper no. 2. University of Warwick: Centre for Research in Ethnic Relations

Owen, D. (1994a) 'Spatial variations in ethnic minority groups populations in Great Britain', *Population Trends*, no. 78, pp. 23–33

Owen, D. (1994b) *Black People in Great Britain: Social and Economic Circumstances*, National Ethnic Minority Data Archive 1991 Census Statistical Paper no. 6. University of Warwick: Centre for Research in Ethnic Relations

Owen, D. (1994c) *South Asian People in Great Britain: Social and Economic Circumstances*, National Ethnic Minority Data Archive 1991 Census Statistical Paper no. 7. University of Warwick: Centre for Research in Ethnic Relations

Owen, D. (1994d) *Chinese People and 'Other' Ethnic Minorities in Great Britain: Social and Economic Circumstances*, National Ethnic Minority Data Archive 1991 Census Statistical Paper no. 8. University of Warwick: Centre for Research in Ethnic Relations

Owen, D. (1995) *Irish-born People in Great Britain*, National Ethnic Minority Data Archive 1991 Census Statistical Paper no. 9. University of Warwick: Centre for Research in Ethnic Relations

Peach, C. (ed.) (1996) *Ethnicity in the 1991 Census. Volume Two: The Ethnic Minority Populations of Great Britain*. London: HMSO

Peach, C. and Winchester, S. (1974) 'Birthplace, ethnicity and the underenumeration of West Indians, Indians and Pakistanis in the Censuses of 1966 and 1971', *New Community*, vol. 3, no. 4, pp. 386–93

Pilgrim, S., Fenton, S., Hughes, T., Hine, C. and Tibbs, N. (1993) *The Bristol Black and Ethnic Minorities Health Survey Report*. Bristol: University of Bristol

Rack, P. (1982) *Race, Culture and Mental Disorder*. London: Tavistock

Ratcliffe, P. (ed.) (1996) *Ethnicity in the 1991 Census. Volume 3: Social Geography and Ethnicity in Britain: Geographical Spread, Spatial Concentration and Internal Migration*. London: HMSO

Robinson, V. (1989) 'Race, space and place: the geographical study of UK ethnic relations 1957–1987', *New Community*, vol. 14, no. 1, pp. 186–97

Rogers, A. (1990) 'Policing mental disorder: controversies, myths and realities', *Social Policy and Administration*, vol. 24, no. 3, pp. 226–36

Rogers, R. (1992) 'Living and dying in the USA: sociodemographic determinants of death among blacks and whites', *Demography*, vol. 29, no. 2, pp. 287–303

Roman, E., Beral, V., Inskip, H., McDowall, M. and Adelstein, A. (1984) 'A comparison of standardized and proportional mortality ratios', *Statistics in Medicine*, vol. 3, pp. 7–14

Rose, G.A. and Blackburn, H. (1986) *Cardiovascular Survey Methods*. Geneva: World Health Organisation

Rudat, K. (1994) *Black and Minority Ethnic Groups in England: Health and Lifestyles*. London: Health Education Authority

Sashidharan, S. and Francis, E. (1993) 'Epidemiology, ethnicity and schizophrenia'. In W.I.U. Ahmad, (ed.) *'Race' and Health in Contemporary Britain*. Buckingham: Open University Press

Sashidharan, S.P. (1993) 'Afro-Caribbeans and schizophrenia: the ethnic vulnerability hypothesis re-examined', *International Review of Psychiatry*, vol. 5, pp. 129–44

Scambler, G. and Higgs, P. (1999) 'Stratification, class and health: class relations and health inequalities in high modernity', *Sociology*, vol. 33, no. 2, pp. 275–96

Scott, A. (1990) *Ideology and the New Social Movements*. London: Unwin Hyman

Senior, P.A. and Bhopal, R. (1994) 'Ethnicity as a variable in epidemiological research', *British Medical Journal*, vol. 309, pp. 327–30

Shaukat, N. and Cruickshank, J. (1993) 'Coronary artery disease: impact upon black and ethnic minority people'. In A. Hopkins and V. Bahl (eds) *Access to Health Care for People from Black and Ethnic Minorities*. London: Royal College of Physicians

Shaukat, N., de Bono, D.P. and Cruickshank, J.K. (1993) 'Clinical features, risk factors and referral delay in British patients of Indian and European origin with angina', *British Medical Journal*, vol. 307, pp. 717–18

Shaukat, N., Lear, J., Fletcher, S., de Bono, D.P. and Woods, K.L. (1997) 'First myocardial infarction in patients of Indian subcontinent and European origin: comparison of risk factors, management, and long term outcome', *British Medical Journal*, vol. 314, pp. 639–42

Sheldon, T.A. and Parker, H. (1992) 'Race and ethnicity in health research', *Journal of Public Health Medicine*, vol. 14, no. 2, pp. 104–110

Simmons, D., Williams, D.R.R. and Powell, M.J. (1989) 'Prevalence of diabetes in a predominantly Asian community: preliminary findings of the Coventry diabetes study', *British Medical Journal*, vol. 298, pp. 18–21

Sloggett, A. and Joshi, H. (1994) 'Higher mortality in deprived areas: community or personal disadvantage?', *British Medical Journal*, vol. 309, pp. 1470–4

Smaje, C. (1995a) 'Ethnic residential concentration and health: evidence for a positive effect?', *Policy and Politics*, vol. 23, no. 3, pp. 251–69

Smaje, C. (1995b) *Health, 'Race' and Ethnicity: Making Sense of the Evidence*. London: King's Fund

Smaje, C. (1996) 'The ethnic patterning of health: new directions for theory and research', *Sociology of Health and Illness*, vol. 18, no. 2, pp. 139–71

Smith, D. (1977) *Racial Disadvantage in Britain*. Harmondsworth: Penguin

Smith, P. (1996) 'Methodological aspects of research amongst ethnic minorities', *Survey Methods Centre Newsletter*, vol. 16, no. 1, pp. 20–4

Smith, P. and Prior, G. (1997) *The Fourth National Survey of Ethnic Minorities: Technical Report*. London: Social and Community Planning Research

Soni Raleigh, V. (1996) 'Suicide patterns and trends in people of Indian subcontinent and Caribbean origin in England and Wales', *Ethnicity and Health*, vol. 1, no. 1, pp. 55–63

Soni Raleigh, V., Bulusu, L. and Balarajan, R. (1990) 'Suicides among immigrants from the Indian subcontinent', *British Journal of Psychiatry*, vol. 156, pp. 46–50

Soni Raleigh, V. and Balarajan, R. (1992a) 'Suicide and self-burning among Indians and West Indians in England and Wales', *British Journal of Psychiatry*, vol. 161, pp. 365–8

Soni Raleigh, V. and Balarajan, R. (1992b) 'Suicide levels and trends among immigrants in England and Wales', *Health Trends*, vol. 24, no. 3, pp. 91–4

Stein, C.E., Fall, C.H., Kumaran, K., Osmond, C., Cox, V. and Barker, D.J. (1996) 'Fetal growth and coronary heart disease in south India', *The Lancet*, vol. 348, pp. 1269–73

Sterling, T., Rosenbaum, W. and Weinkam, J. (1993) 'Income, race and mortality', *Journal of the National Medical Association*, vol. 85, no. 12, pp. 906–11

Sugarman, P.A. and Craufurd, D. (1994) 'Schizophrenia in the Afro-Caribbean Community', *British Journal of Psychiatry*, vol. 164, pp. 474–80

Syme, S., Marmot, M., Kagan, H. and Rhoads, G. (1975) 'Epidemiologic studies of CHD and stroke in Japanese men living in Japan, Hawaii and California', *American Journal of Epidemiology*, vol. 102, pp. 477–480

Thomas, R. and Purdon, S. (1994) 'Using the results of the 1991 Census question on limiting long-term illness', *Survey Methods Centre Newsletter*, vol. 14, no. 2, pp. 7–13

Townsend, P. and Davidson, N. (1982) *Inequalities in Health (the Black Report)*. Harmondsworth: Penguin

Townsend, P., Phillimore, P. and Beattie, A. (1988) *Health and Deprivation: Inequality and the North*. London: Routledge

Vågerö, D. and Illsley, R. (1995) 'Explaining health inequalities: beyond Black and Barker', *European Sociological Review*, vol. 11, no. 3, pp. 219–39

van Os, J., Castle, D.J., Takei, N., Der, G. and Murray, R.M. (1996) 'Psychotic illnes in ethnic minorities: clarification from the 1991 Census', *Psychological Medicine*, vol. 26, pp. 203–8

Virdee, S. (1995) *Racial Violence and Harassment*. London: Policy Studies Institute

Virdee, S. (1997) 'Racial harassment'. In T. Modood, R. Berthoud, J. Lakey, J. Nazroo, P. Smith, S. Virdee and S. Beishon, *Ethnic Minorities in Britain: Diversity and Disadvantage*. London: Policy Studies Institute

Ware, J.E. and Sherbourne, C.D. (1992) 'The MOS 36-Item Short-Form Health Survey (SF–36). 1. Conceptual framework and item selection', *Medical Care*, vol. 30, no. 6, pp. 473–83

White, A., Nicolaas, G., Foster, K., Browne, F. and Carey, S. (1993) *Health Survey for England 1991*. London: HMSO

WHO (World Health Organisation) (1992) *International Classification of Mental and Behavioural Disorders*. Geneva: World Health Organisation

Wild, S. and McKeigue, P. (1997) 'Cross sectional analysis of mortality by country of birth in England and Wales', *British Medical Journal*, vol. 314, pp. 705–10

Wilkinson, P., Sayer, J., Koorithottumkal, L., Grundy, C., Marchant, B., Kopelman, P. and Timmis, A.D. (1996) 'Comparison of case fatality in south Asian and white patients after acute myocardial infarction: observational study', *British Medical Journal*, vol. 312, pp. 1330–3

Wilkinson, R. (1994) *Unfair Shares*. Ilford: Barnardo's

Wilkinson, R.G. (1996) *Unhealthy Societies: The Afflictions of Inequality*. London: Routledge

Williams, D.R., Lavizzo-Mourey, R. and Warren, R.C. (1994) 'The concept of race and health status in America', *Public Health Reports*, vol. 109, no. 1, pp. 26–41

Williams, R. (1993) 'Health and length of residence among South Asians in Glasgow: a study controlling for age', *Journal of Public Health Medicine*, vol. 15, no. 1, pp. 52–60

Williams, R., Bhopal, R. and Hunt, K. (1993) 'Health of a Punjabi ethnic minority in Glasgow: a comparison with the general population', *Journal of Epidemiology and Community Health*, vol. 47, pp. 96–102

Williams, R., Eley, S., Hunt, K. and Bhatt, S. (1997) 'Has psychological distress among UK South Asians been under-estimated? A comparison of three measures in the west of Scotland population', *Ethnicity and Health*, vol. 2, pp. 21–29

Williams, R. and Hunt, K. (1997) 'Psychological distress among British South Asians: the contribution of stressful situations and subcultural differences in the West of Scotland Twenty–07 Study', *Psychological Medicine*, vol. 27, pp. 1173–81

Wing, J.K., Cooper, J.E. and Sartorius, N. (1974) *Measurement and Classification of Psychiatric Symptoms*. Cambridge: Cambridge University Press

# Appendix A: Health Questionnaire

E2/H 26

## HEALTH

CARD 29
(2914-17)

H1   I would now like to ask you about your health and the use you make of health services.
Please think back over the last 12 months about how your health has been. Compared to people of
your own age, would you say that your health has on the whole been...READ OUT...

| | | |
|---|---|---|
| ...excellent, | 1 | 2918 |
| good, | 2 | |
| fair, | 3 | |
| poor, | 4 | |
| or very poor? | 5 | |
| Can't say | 8 | |

H2a)   Do you have any long-standing illness, disability or infirmity? By long-standing I mean anything
that has troubled you over a period of time that is likely to affect you over a period of time?

| | | | |
|---|---|---|---|
| Yes | 1 ASK b) | | 2919 |
| No | 2 GO TO H3 | | |

IF YES

H2b)   What is the matter with you?                                                    2920-39
TRY TO OBTAIN A MEDICAL DIAGNOSIS OR ESTABLISH MAIN SYMPTOMS

c)   INTERVIEWER CODE

| | | |
|---|---|---|
| Complaint on Reference Card RA | 1 | 2940 |
| All others | 2 | |

IF ILLNESS/DISABILITY/INFIRMITY

d)   Does this problem limit the kind of paid work that you can do (or could do if wanted to)?

| | | |
|---|---|---|
| Yes | 1 | 2941 |
| No | 2 | |

H3   Can I check, are you registered as a disabled person, either with Social Services or with a green
card?

| | | |
|---|---|---|
| Yes | 1 | 2942 |
| No | 2 | |

Unsure          8

H4      Are you currently taking or using any medicines, pills, ointments or injections of any kind?
        INCLUDES "ALTERNATIVE" HEALTH REMEDIES

                                                        Yes          1 ASK H5          2943
                                                        No           2 GO TO H6

IF YES AT H4

H5a)    Please could you tell me what they are.                                      2944–71
        PROBE FOR FULL DETAILS OF MEDICINES, PILLS, OINTMENTS, AND
        INJECTIONS/IMPLANTS. ASK TO SEE BOTTLES IF POSSIBLE

        MEDICINES: _____

        _____

        _____

        PILLS:     _____

        _____

        OINTMENTS: _____

        _____

        INJECTIONS/_____
        IMPLANTS:  _____

        _____

        _____

b)      INTERVIEWER CODE
                                Medication on Reference Card RB          1          2972
                                            All others          2

H6      Do you now have or have you ever had any of the following conditions?          CARD 30

        READ OUT AND RING ONE CODE FOR EACH

                                                        Yes          No
        High blood pressure, sometimes called hypertension
        (apart from during pregnancy)?                   1           2          3014
        A stroke?                                        1           2          3015
        Diabetes?                                        1           2          3016
        Angina?                                          1           2          3017
        A heart attack – including a heart murmur, a
        damaged heart or a rapid heart?                  1           2          3018

H7a)    CHECK H6 AND RECORD:
                                        Has or had diabetes          1 ASK b)          3019
                                                Others          2 GO TO H8
        IF HAS OR HAD DIABETES
b)      Do you attend a diabetes treatment clinic?
                                                        Yes          1          3020
                                                        No           2

H8a)    INTERVIEWER CHECK A1a) AND RECORD:
                                Respondent aged 40 or over          1 CHECK b)          3021
                                Respondent aged under 40          2 GO TO H10

b)      INTERVIEWER CHECK H6 AND RECORD:

|  |  |  |
|---|---|---|
| Respondent reported no heart problems (CODE 2 FOR ANGINA AND HEART ATTACK) | 1 ASK H9 | 3022 |
| Respondent reported heart problems | 2 GO TO H10 | |

H9a)    Have you ever had any pain or discomfort in your chest?

|  |  |  |
|---|---|---|
| Yes | 1 ASK b) | 3023 |
| No | 2 GO TO H10 | |

IF YES

H9b)    Have you ever had a severe pain across the front of your chest lasting for more than half an hour?

|  |  |  |
|---|---|---|
| Yes | 1 ASK c) | 3024 |
| No | 2 GO TO H10 | |

IF YES

c)      Did you see a doctor because of this pain?

|  |  |  |
|---|---|---|
| Yes | 1 ASK d) | 3025 |
| No | 2 GO TO H10 | |

IF YES

d)      What did the doctor say?

|  |  |  |
|---|---|---|
| Angina | 1 | 3026 |
| Heart attack | 2 | |
| Did not say | 3 | |
| Other (SPECIFY) _____ | 4 | |

ALL

H10   The following questions are about activities you might do during a typical day.

    a)    Does your health limit you when you take part in ...

READ OUT AND CODE ONE FOR EACH IN GRID AT a)
IF "YES" AT (a), ASK b)

    b)    How much does your health limit you in – (ACTIVITY) - a lot or a little?

RING ONE CODE FOR EACH IN GRID UNDER (b)

|  | (a) | | (b) | | | |
|---|---|---|---|---|---|---|
|  | | | Wouldn't | Limited | Limited | |
|  | | | ever | a | a | |
|  | Yes | No | do | lot | little | |
| ...vigorous activities, such as running, lifting heavy objects or participating in strenuous sports? | 1 | 2 | 3 | 1 | 2 | 3027–28 |
| ...moderate activities such as moving a table, pushing a vacuum cleaner, bowling or playing golf? | 1 | 2 | 3 | 1 | 2 | 3029–30 |
| ...lifting or carrying groceries? | 1 | 2 | 3 | 1 | 2 | 3031–32 |
| ...climbing several flights of stairs? | 1 | 2 | 3 | 1 | 2 | 3033–34 |
| ...climbing one flight of stairs? | 1 | 2 | 3 | 1 | 2 | 3035–36 |
| ...bending, kneeling or stooping? | 1 | 2 | 3 | 1 | 2 | 3037–38 |
| ...walking more than a mile? | 1 | 2 | 3 | 1 | 2 | 3039–40 |
| ...walking half a mile? | 1 | 2 | 3 | 1 | 2 | 3041–42 |
| ...walking 100 yards? | 1 | 2 | 3 | 1 | 2 | 3043–44 |
| ...bathing or dressing yourself? | 1 | 2 | 3 | 1 | 2 | 3045–46 |
|  | | | | | | (3047–50) |

H11a)  Have you had attacks of wheezing or whistling in your chest at any time in the last 12 months?

|  | | |
|---|---|---|
| Yes | 1 | 3051 |
| No | 2 | |

b)  Have you ever had attacks of shortness of breath with wheezing?

|  | | |
|---|---|---|
| Yes | 1 ASK c) | 3052 |
| No | 2 GO TO H12 | |

IF YES

H11c)  Is your breathing absolutely normal between attacks?

|  | | |
|---|---|---|
| Yes | 1 | 3053 |
| No | 2 | |

d)  Have you at any time in the last twelve months been woken at night by an attack of shortness of breath?

|  | | |
|---|---|---|
| Yes | 1 | 3054 |
| No | 2 | |

H12a)  Do you usually bring up any phlegm from your chest first thing in the morning in the winter?

|  | | |
|---|---|---|
| Yes | 1 GO TO c) | 3055 |
| No | 2 ASK b) | |

IF NO

b)  Do you usually bring up any phlegm from your chest during the day or night in the winter?

|  | | |
|---|---|---|
| Yes | 1 ASK c) | 3056 |
| No | 2 GO TO H13 | |

IF YES

c)  Do you bring up phlegm like this on most days for as much as three months each year?

|  | | |
|---|---|---|
| Yes | 1 | 3057 |
| No | 2 | |

H13a)  Would you say that for your height you are...
READ OUT...

|  | | |
|---|---|---|
| ...about the right weight, | 1 | 3058 |
| too heavy, | 2 | |
| or too light? | 3 | |
| Can't say | 8 | |

b)  Have you ever seriously tried to lose weight?

|  | | |
|---|---|---|
| Yes | 1 | 3059 |
| No | 2 | |

H14a)  Have you ever smoked a cigarette (IF ASIAN: or Bidi), a cigar or a pipe?

|  | | |
|---|---|---|
| Yes | 1 ASK b) | 3060 |
| No | 2 GO TO H15 | |

IF YES

b)  Do you smoke cigarettes (IF ASIAN: or Bidis) at all nowadays?

|  | | |
|---|---|---|
| Yes | 1 GO TO e) | 3061 |
| No | 2 ASK c) | |

IF NO

c)  Have you ever smoked cigarettes (or Bidis)?

|  | | |
|---|---|---|
| Yes | 1 ASK d) | 3062 |
| No | 2 GO TO H15 | |

IF YES
H14d) Did you smoke cigarettes (or Bidis) regularly or occasionally? By regularly, I mean at least one cigarette (or Bidi) a day.

|  |  |  |
|---|---|---|
| Regularly | 1 | 3063 |
| Occasionally | 2 GO TO H15 | |
| Never really smoked, just tried it once or twice | 3 | |

## CURRENT SMOKERS

e) About how many cigarettes (or Bidis) a day do you usually smoke on weekdays?

| | | |
|---|---|---|
| WRITE IN NUMBER: | | 3064–65 |
| OR CODE: Can't say | 98 | |

f) And about how many cigarettes (or Bidis) a day do you usually smoke at weekends?

| | | |
|---|---|---|
| WRITE IN NUMBER: | | 3066–67 |
| OR CODE: Can't say | 98 | |

H15a) Have you ever had paan (betel)?

| | | |
|---|---|---|
| Yes | 1 ASK b) | 3068 |
| No | 2 GO TO H16 | |

IF YES
b) Do you have paan (betel) nowadays?
IF YES:
Do you have it regularly or just occasionally?

| | | |
|---|---|---|
| Yes, regularly | 1 | 3069 |
| Yes, occasionally | 2 | |
| No | 3 | |

H16 How often, if ever, do you drink alcohol?                                    CARD 31

| | | |
|---|---|---|
| Once a week or more often | 1 ASK H17 | 3114 |
| Less often than once a week | 2 | |
| Never drink alcohol | 3 GO TO H18 | |

IF DRINK ALCOHOL
H17 Thinking about the last three months only, have you at any time
...READ OUT AND CODE YES OR NO FOR EACH ...

| | Yes | No | Can't say | |
|---|---|---|---|---|
| ... found that your hands were shaking in the morning after drinking the previous night? | 1 | 2 | 8 | 3115 |
| ... had a drink first thing in the morning to steady your nerves or get rid of a hangover? | 1 | 2 | 8 | 3116 |

H18 The next few questions are about how you feel in yourself - your general well-being.
a) Have you noticed that you've been getting tired in the past month?

| | | |
|---|---|---|
| Yes | 1 GO TO c) | 3117 |
| No | 2 ASK b) | |

IF NO
b) During the past month, have you felt you've been lacking in energy?

| | | |
|---|---|---|
| Yes | 1 ASK c) | 3118 |
| No | 2 GO TO H19 | |

IF TIRED OR LACKING IN ENERGY
c) Do you know why you have been feeling (tired/lacking in energy)?

| | | |
|---|---|---|
| Yes | 1 ASK d) | 3119 |
| No | 2 GO TO H19 | |

IF YES

d)    SHOW CARD HA. What is the main reason? Please choose from this card.
      CODE ALL THAT APPLY

|  | | |
|---|---|---|
| Problems with sleep | 1 | 3120–26 |
| Medication | 2 | |
| Physical illness | 3 | |
| Working too hard (inc. housework, looking after baby) | 4 | |
| Stress, worry or some other psychological reason | 5 | |
| Physical exercise | 6 | |
| Other (SPECIFY)_____ | 7 | |

ALL

H19a)  In the past month, have you been having problems with trying to get to sleep or with getting back
       to sleep if you were woken?

|  | | |
|---|---|---|
| Yes | 1 | 3127 |
| No | 2 | |

b)     Has sleeping more than you usually do been a problem for you in the last month?

|  | | |
|---|---|---|
| Yes | 1 | 3128 |
| No | 2 | |

c)     INTERVIEWER CHECK a) AND b) AND RECORD:
       Respondent has sleep problems

|  | | |
|---|---|---|
| ('Yes' AT a) AND/OR b)) | 1 ASK H20 | 3129 |
| Respondent does not have sleep problems | 2 GO TO H21 | |

IF SLEEP PROBLEMS

H20a)  Do you know why you are having problems with your sleep?

|  | | |
|---|---|---|
| Yes | 1 ASK b) | 3130 |
| No | 2 GO TO H21 | |

IF YES

b)     SHOW CARD HB. What is the main reason for these problems?
       Please choose from this card. CODE ALL THAT APPLY

|  | | |
|---|---|---|
| Noise | 01 | 3131–48 |
| Shift work/too busy to sleep | 02 | |
| Illness/discomfort | 03 | |
| Worry/thinking | 04 | |
| Needing to go to the toilet | 05 | |
| Wake to do something (e.g. look after baby) | 06 | |
| Tired | 07 | |
| Medication | 08 | |
| Other (SPECIFY) _____ | 09 | (3149) |

ALL

H21a)  Almost everyone becomes sad, miserable or depressed at times.
       Have you had a spell of feeling sad, miserable or depressed in the past month?

|  | | |
|---|---|---|
| Yes | 1 ASK b) | 3150 |
| No | 2 GO TO c) | |

IF YES

b)     Have you had such a spell in the past week?

|  | | |
|---|---|---|
| Yes | 1 | 3151 |
| No | 2 | |

c) During the past month, have you been able to enjoy or take an interest in things as much as you usually do?

| | | |
|---|---|---|
| Yes | 1 GO TO e) | 3152 |
| No/No enjoyment or interest | 2 ASK d) | |

IF NO

d) Have you felt unable to enjoy or take an interest in things during the past week?

| | | |
|---|---|---|
| Yes, unable to take an interest in things | 1 | 3153 |
| No | 2 | |

e) INTERVIEWER CHECK:

| | | |
|---|---|---|
| 'Yes' AT (b) OR AT (d) | 1 ASK H22 | 3154 |
| Others | 2 GO TO H26 | |

IN QUESTIONS H22 TO H24, READ 'depressed'
    IF RESPONDENT SAID 'Yes' TO b); READ "UNABLE TO TAKE AN INTEREST IN THINGS"
    FOR THE REMAINDER
    IF DEPRESSED/UNABLE TO TAKE INTEREST

H22a) Since last... (DAY OF WEEK)... on how many days have you felt depressed (unable to take an interest in things)?

| | | |
|---|---|---|
| 4 days or more | 1 | 3155 |
| 2 to 3 days | 2 | |
| 1 day | 3 | |
| Can't say | 8 | |

b) Have you felt depressed (unable to enjoy or take an interest in things) for more than 3 hours in total on any day in the past week?

| | | |
|---|---|---|
| Yes | 1 | 3156 |
| No | 2 | |

H23a) SHOW CARD HC. What sort of things made you feel depressed (unable to enjoy or take an interest in things) in the past week? Can you choose from this card?
RING AS MANY CODES AS APPLY IN COLUMN (a)

| | (a) | (b) Main Thing | |
|---|---|---|---|
| Members of the family | 01 | 01 | (a) |
| Relationship with spouse/partner | 02 | 02 | 3157–76 |
| Relationships with friends | 03 | 03 | |
| Housing | 04 | 04 | (b) |
| Money/bills | 05 | 05 | 3177–78 |
| Own physical health (inc. pregnancy) | 06 | 06 | |
| Own mental health | 07 | 07 | |
| Work or lack of work (inc. student) | 08 | 08 | |
| Legal difficulties | 09 | 09 | |
| Political issues/the news | 10 | 10 | |
| Harassment | 11 | 11 | |
| Other (SPECIFY) _____ | 12 | 12 | |
| Can't say | 98 | 98 | |

IF 2+ ANSWERS AT a), ASK b)

b) What was the main thing that made you feel like this?
RING ONE CODE ONLY ABOVE IN COLUMN (b)

c)    In the past week when you felt depressed (unable to enjoy or take an interest in things), did you ever become happier when something nice happened, or when you were in company?

|  |  | CARD 32 |
|---|---|---|
| Yes | 1 | 3214 |
| No | 2 | (3215) |

H23d) How long have you been feeling depressed (unable to take an interest in things) as you have described?

| | | |
|---|---|---|
| less than 2 weeks | 1 | 3216 |
| 2 weeks but less than 6 months | 2 | |
| 6 months but less than 1 year | 3 | |
| 1 year but less than 2 years | 4 | |
| 2 years or more | 5 | |

H24a) In the past week were these feelings worse in the morning or in the evening, or did this make no difference?

| | | |
|---|---|---|
| Worse in the morning | 1 | 3217 |
| Worse in the evening | 2 | |
| No difference/Other | 3 | |

b)    When you have felt sad, miserable or depressed (unable to take an interest in things) in the past week, have you been so restless that you couldn't sit still?

| | | |
|---|---|---|
| Yes | 1 | 3218 |
| No | 2 | |

c)    And have you been doing things more slowly, for example, walking more slowly?

| | | |
|---|---|---|
| Yes | 1 | 3219 |
| No | 2 | |

H24d) Have you been less talkative than normal?

| | | |
|---|---|---|
| Yes | 1 | 3220 |
| No | 2 | |

e)    Again, thinking about the past seven days, have you on at least one occasion felt guilty or blamed yourself when things went wrong when it hasn't been your fault?

| | | |
|---|---|---|
| Yes | 1 | 3221 |
| No | 2 | |

f)    During the past week, have you been feeling you are not as good as other people?

| | | |
|---|---|---|
| Yes | 1 | 3222 |
| No | 2 | |

g)    Have you felt hopeless at all during the past week, for instance about your future?

| | | |
|---|---|---|
| Yes | 1 | 3223 |
| No | 2 | |

h)    INTERVIEWER CHECK e), f) AND g) AND RECORD:

| | | |
|---|---|---|
| 'Yes' e), f) OR g) | 1 ASK H25 | 3224 |
| Others | 2 GO TO H26 | |

IF CODE 1 AT H24h)

H25a) In the past week, have you felt that life isn't worth living?

| | | |
|---|---|---|
| Yes | 1 ASK b) | 3225 |
| Yes, but not in the past week | 2 GO TO H26 d) | |
| No | 3 | |

IF YES

b)  In the past week, have you thought of committing suicide?

|  |  |  |
|---|---|---|
| Yes | 1 ASK b) | 3226 |
| Yes, but not in the past week | 2 GO TO H26 d) | |
| No | 3 | |

IF YES

c)  Have you talked to your doctor about these thoughts (of committing suicide)?

|  |  |  |
|---|---|---|
| Yes | 1 GO TO H26 | 3227 |
| No | 2 READ d) | |

IF NO

d)  (You have said that you thought about committing suicide). Since this is a very serious matter, it is most important that you talk to your doctor about these thoughts

ALL

H26  (Thank you for answering those questions on how you have been feeling). I would now like to ask you a few questions about worries you might have.

a)  Have you been feeling anxious or nervous in the past month?

|  |  |  |
|---|---|---|
| Yes | 1 | 3228 |
| No | 2 | |

b)  In the past month, did you ever find your muscles felt tense or that you couldn't relax?

|  |  |  |
|---|---|---|
| Yes | 1 | 3229 |
| No | 2 | |

H26c)  Some people have phobias; they get nervous or uncomfortable about particular things or situations when there is no real danger.
In the past month, have you felt anxious, nervous or tense about any particular things or situations when there was no real danger?
IF NECESSARY: For example, you may get nervous when speaking or eating in front of strangers, when you are far from home or in crowded rooms, or you may have a fear of heights. You may become nervous at the sight of things like blood or spiders.

|  |  |  |
|---|---|---|
| Yes | 1 ASK H27 | 3230 |
| No | 2 GO TO H28 | |

IF YES

H27  SHOW CARD HD. Can you look at this card and tell me which of the situations or things listed made you the most anxious in the past month?
CODE ALL THAT APPLY

|  |  |  |
|---|---|---|
| Crowds or public places, including travelling alone or being far from home | 1 | 3231–36 |
| Enclosed spaces | 2 | |
| Social situations, including eating or speaking in public, being watched or stared at | 3 | |
| The sight of blood or injury | 4 | |
| Any specific single cause including insects, spiders and heights | 5 | |
| Other things | 6 | |

H28a)  INTERVIEWER CHECK H26a), b) AND c) AND CODE FIRST TO APPLY

|  |  |  |
|---|---|---|
| 'Yes' AT a) OR b) | 1 ASK b) | 3237 |
| 'Yes' AT c) | 2 GO TO c) | |
| Others | 3 GO TO H29 | |

IF CODE 1 AT a)

H28b) Which, if any, of the following symptoms did you have when you felt anxious?

READ OUT AND CODE YES OR NO FOR EACH

| | Yes | No | |
|---|---|---|---|
| Heart racing or pounding | 1 | 2 | 3238 |
| Hands sweating or shaking | 1 | 2 | 3239 |
| Feeling dizzy | 1 | 2 | 3240 |
| Difficulty getting your breath | 1 | 2 | 3241 |
| Butterflies in stomach | 1 | 2 | 3242 |
| Dry mouth | 1 | 2 | 3243 |
| Nausea or feeling as though you wanted to vomit | 1 | 2 | 3244 |

IF CODE 1 OR 2 AT a)

c) Thinking about the last month, did your anxiety or tension ever get so bad that you got into a panic, for instance, make you feel that you might collapse or lose control unless you did something about it?

| | | |
|---|---|---|
| Yes | 1 | 3245 |
| No | 2 | |

ALL

H29 Over the past year, have there been times when you felt very happy indeed without a break for days on end?

| | | |
|---|---|---|
| Yes | 1 ASK H30 | 3246 |
| Unsure | 2 GO TO H31 | |
| No | 3 | |

IF YES

H30a) Was there an obvious reason for this?

| | | |
|---|---|---|
| Yes | 1 | 3247 |
| Unsure | 2 | |
| No | 3 | |

b) Did your relatives or friends think it was strange or complain about it?

| | | |
|---|---|---|
| Yes | 1 | 3248 |
| Unsure | 2 | |
| No | 3 | |

ALL

H31a) Over the past year, have you ever felt that your thoughts were directly interfered with or controlled by some outside force or person?

| | | |
|---|---|---|
| Yes | 1 ASK b) | 3249 |
| Unsure | 2 GO TO H32 | |
| No | 3 | |

IF YES

H31b) Did this come about in a way that many people would find hard to believe, for instance, through telepathy?

| | | |
|---|---|---|
| Yes | 1 | 3250 |
| Unsure | 2 | |
| No | 3 | |

H32a) Over the past year, have there been times when you felt that people were against you?

| | | |
|---|---|---|
| Yes | 1 ASK b) | 3251 |
| Unsure | 2 GO TO H33 | |
| No | 3 | |

IF YES

b)    Have there been times when you felt that people were deliberately acting to harm you or your
      interests?

|           |   |      |
|-----------|---|------|
| Yes       | 1 | 3252 |
| Unsure    | 2 |      |
| No        | 3 |      |

c)    Have there been times you felt that a group of people were plotting to cause you serious harm or
      injury?

|           |   |      |
|-----------|---|------|
| Yes       | 1 | 3253 |
| Unsure    | 2 |      |
| No        | 3 |      |

H33   Over the past year, have there been times when you felt that something strange was going on?

|        |              |      |
|--------|--------------|------|
| Yes    | 1 ASK H34    | 3254 |
| Unsure | 2 GO TO H35  |      |
| No     | 3            |      |

IF YES

H34   Did you feel it was so strange that other people would find it very hard to believe?

|        |   |      |
|--------|---|------|
| Yes    | 1 | 3255 |
| Unsure | 2 |      |
| No     | 3 |      |

ALL

H35a)  Over the past year, have there been times when you heard or saw things that other people
       couldn't?

|        |              |      |
|--------|--------------|------|
| Yes    | 1 ASK b)     | 3256 |
| Unsure | 2 GO TO H36  |      |
| No     | 3            |      |

IF YES

b)    Did you at any time hear voices saying quite a few words or sentences when there was no one
      around that might account for it?

|        |   |      |
|--------|---|------|
| Yes    | 1 | 3257 |
| Unsure | 2 |      |
| No     | 3 |      |

H36   INTERVIEWER RECORD ANY COMMENTS MADE SPONTANEOUSLY WHICH WOULD HELP
      INTERPRETATION OF ANSWERS H29–H35

ALL

H37   Over the past month, approximately how many times have you talked to, or visited a GP or family
      doctor about your own health? Please do not include any visits to a hospital, or visits you made
      while abroad.

|               |              |      |
|---------------|--------------|------|
| One or two    | 1            | 3258 |
| Three to five | 2            |      |
| Six to ten    | 3 ASK H38    |      |
| More than ten | 4            |      |
| None          | 5 GO TO H39  |      |
| Can't say     | 8            |      |

IF VISITED IN PAST MONTH

H38a)  Did the doctor speak a language you could clearly understand?

|                        |              |      |
|------------------------|--------------|------|
| Yes                    | 1 GO TO H39  | 3259 |
| No                     | 2 ASK b)     |      |
| Some did, some didn't  | 3            |      |

IF NO/SOME DID AND SOME DIDN'T

H38b)  How did you manage to communicate to the doctor(s) who did not speak a language
you could understand?                                                                                    3260–71
PROBE FULLY. RECORD VERBATIM

c)  Do you think the doctor understood you?                                              CARD 33

| | | |
|---|---|---|
| Yes | 1 | 3314 |
| No | 2 | |

H39a)  In the past twelve months have you spoken to a GP or family doctor on your own behalf, either in
person or by telephone, about being anxious or depressed or a mental, nervous or emotional
problem?

| | | |
|---|---|---|
| Yes | 1 ASK b) | 3315 |
| No | 2 GO TO H40 | |

IF YES

b)  What did the doctor say was the matter with you?                                       3316–31
TRY AND OBTAIN A MEDICAL DIAGNOSIS OR ESTABLISH SYMPTOMS

c)  INTERVIEWER CODE

| | | |
|---|---|---|
| Complaint on Reference Card RA | 1 | 3332 |
| All others | 2 | |

ALL

H40a)  In the last 12 months, that is since ...(MONTH) 1992/1993 have you had any kind of accident as a
result of which you saw a doctor or went to hospital?

| | | |
|---|---|---|
| Yes | 1 ASK b) | 3333 |
| No | 2 GO TO H41 | |

IF YES

b)  Have you had more than one accident, in the last year? IF YES: How many?

| | | |
|---|---|---|
| One only | 1 | 3334 |
| Two | 2 | |
| Three | 3 | |
| Four or more | 4 | |

ASK c) AND d) FOR EACH ACCIDENT IN PAST
12 MONTHS STARTING WITH MOST RECENT

c)  In which year and month did ... (accident) happen?
ENTER YEAR AND MONTH IN COLUMN (c) IN GRID

d)  Where did this accident happen? PROMPT AS NECESSARY AND
RING ONE CODE IN COLUMN (d) ON GRID

| | (c) | | (d) | | | | | |
|---|---|---|---|---|---|---|---|---|
| | When happened | | Where accident happened | | | | | |
| Accident | Year | Month | Sports facilities | Workplace | Home/ garden | School/ College | Motor/ vehicle | Road/ pavement | Other |
| (SPECIFY) | | | | | | | | |
| Most recent | 1 | 2 | 3 | 4 | 5 | 6 | 7_____ | 3335–39 |
| 2nd most recent | 1 | 2 | 3 | 4 | 5 | 6 | 7_____ | 3340–44 |
| 3rd most recent | 1 | 2 | 3 | 4 | 5 | 6 | 7_____ | 3345–49 |
| 4th most recent | 1 | 2 | 3 | 4 | 5 | 6 | 7_____ | 3350–54 |
| 5th most recent | 1 | 2 | 3 | 4 | 5 | 6 | 7_____ | 3355–59 |

H41a) In the last 12 months, that is since ... (MONTH) ... 1992/1993, have you been in hospital or in a clinic as an in-patient overnight or longer?
INCLUDE CHILDBIRTH

|  |  |  |  |
|---|---|---|---|
|  | Yes | 1 ASK b) | 3360 |
|  | No | 2 GO TO H44 |  |

IF YES

b) Since ... (MONTH) ... 1992/1993, in all, how many days have you spent in hospital or in a clinic as an in-patient?

|  |  |  |
|---|---|---|
| WRITE IN NO. OF DAYS: |  | 3361–62 |
| OR CODE: Can't remember/Can't say | 98 |  |

c) Did you receive any assistance from a hospital linkworker, advocate or interpreter?

|  |  |  |
|---|---|---|
| Yes | 1 | 3363 |
| No | 2 |  |

d) Was (were) your hospital stay(s) free under the NHS or paid for privately?

|  |  |  |
|---|---|---|
| All free under the NHS | 1 | 3364 |
| All paid for privately | 2 |  |
| Some NHS/some private | 3 |  |
| Can't say | 8 |  |

H42 INTERVIEWER CHECK A1a) AND RECORD:

|  |  |  |
|---|---|---|
| Respondent is female and under 45 | 1 ASK H43 | 3365 |
| Others | 2 GO TO H44 |  |

IF CODE 1 AT H42

H43 Were any of these hospital stays for child-birth?

|  |  |  |
|---|---|---|
| Yes, all | 1 | 3366 |
| Yes, some | 2 |  |
| No | 3 |  |

ALL

H44a) When attending your GP or hospital, would you prefer to be seen by a doctor of - (ETHNIC ORIGIN) -origin?

|  |  |  |
|---|---|---|
| Yes | 1 ASK b) | 3367 |
| No | 2 |  |
| Depends | 3 GO TO H46 |  |
| Can't say | 8 |  |

IF YES

b) Why is that?                                                                                  3368–79
PROBE FULLY AND RECORD VERBATIM

H45 NOT USED

H46 When visiting a GP or hospital, do you prefer to be seen by a...                CARD (3414–25)
READ OUT...

|  |  |  |
|---|---|---|
| ...female doctor, | 1 | 3426 |
| a male doctor, | 2 |  |
| or doesn't it matter to you? | 3 |  |
| (Can't say) | 8 |  |

ALL

H47a)  Finally, here is a list of some health and welfare services. Please tell me for each service, whether
       it is something you have made use of in the last 12 months, that is since - (MONTH) – in last
       year?
       READ OUT AND RING ONE CODE FOR EACH IN GRID AT (a)
       b) ASK (b) FOR EACH SERVICE USED
       Thinking of - (SERVICE) - , was this provided by the NHS or Social Services, or was it provided by
       a private or voluntary agency?
       RING ONE CODE FOR EACH IN GRID IN (b)

|  | (a) Used | | | (b) Provider | | | |
| --- | --- | --- | --- | --- | --- | --- | --- |
|  | Yes | No | Unsure | NHS | Social services | Private/ voluntary | Unknown agency |
| Dentist | 1 | 2 | 8 | 1 | 2 | 3 | 8 | 3427–28 |
| Physiotherapist | 1 | 2 | 8 | 1 | 2 | 3 | 8 | 3429–30 |
| Psychotherapist | 1 | 2 | 8 | 1 | 2 | 3 | 8 | 3431–32 |
| Social Worker or Welfare Officer | 1 | 2 | 8 | 1 | 2 | 3 | 8 | 3433–34 |
| Alternative medical practitioner (e.g. Hakim, homeopath, osteopath) | 1 | 2 | 8 | 1 | 2 | 3 | 8 | 3435–36 |
| Health Visitor or District Nurse | 1 | 2 | 8 | 1 | 2 | 3 | 8 | 3437–38 |
| Home Help | 1 | 2 | 8 | 1 | 2 | 3 | 8 | 3439–40 |
| (IF AGED 65+) Meals on wheels | 1 | 2 | 8 | 1 | 2 | 3 | 8 | 3441–42 |
| Some other health or Welfare service | 1 | 2 | 8 | 1 | 2 | 3 | 8 | 3443–44 |